META ANATOMY

MetaAnatomy

Anatomy of a Yogi

VOLUME ONE INTRODUCTIONS

-by -

Kristin Leal

Preface

I still get giddy every time I get the chance to talk to someone about his or her magnificent form! As a student of the body for the last 20 years, I am still amazed at the hidden gems and the new information that I continue to learn. My intent in launching MetaAnatomy was to explore the dynamic beauty and poetry of who you are. The prefix Meta, like in the words metaphysical or metacarpals, means beyond, and MetaAnatomy is my attempt to go beyond our often limited concepts of our own form. Combining the physical and energetic anatomies helps us to form a richer view and experience of ourselves. My hope is that this will bring about a celebration of our differences and, ultimately, an honoring of our connectedness.

In this book, MetaAnatomy Volume One, I want to introduce you to your physical form. While I have directed these writings towards students and teachers of yoga, I firmly believe that it includes information that everyone should know. Please keep in mind that this is just an introduction to some of the tissues of the body. In the interest of brevity and comprehension, only certain bones, joints, and muscles have been illuminated. I have tried to distill what can be the overwhelming topic of human anatomy into fun-size bites. In this attempt, some aspects have been simplified and generalized - hopefully without losing their accuracy and importance. Many teachers over the years have informed this work, shaped my ideas, and fired up my passion for the body. To them, I am eternally grateful.

I would like to express my profound gratitude to my first teachers, Christopher and Marianne Leal (otherwise known as Mom and Dad). Their unyielding support and confidence in me continues to shape who I am and everything I do. To Tracy and Tommy Cecil, whose humor, love, and fine dining keeps me going. To Andrea Borrero, for believing in MetaAnatomy, being the catalyst for its development, and for her endless patience with my gazillion questions. To my family at ISHTA Yoga, especially Alan, Sarah, and Satya Finger, for their constant inspiration and refinement of my work. To my friends and teachers Adrienne Burke, Jill Camera, and Tania Varela-Ibarra, whose late night philosophy talks spark my passion for this work. To Kimberly Wilson, for being a shining example of how to share your passion with the world and for helping me to navigate the world of publishing and promotion. To Maria Alcira Gonzalez, for her brilliant creativity and design of this book. And last, but certainly not least, Rebecca Baczek and Jessica DeMers Puk at BrInk Editing, and Dr. Rajiv Arapurakal for their support and keen editor eyes.

Table of Contents

Chapter 1

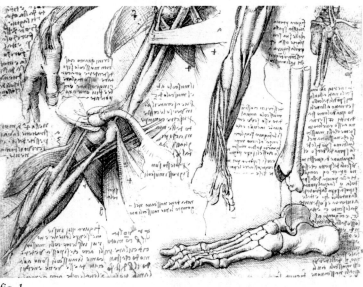

fig. 1

Hello? Is It Me You're Looking For?

PROPER INTRODUCTIONS

> "Dispel from your mind the thought that an understanding of the human body in every aspect of its structure can be given in words..."
>
> - LEONARDO DA VINCI

Oh my goodness! Where are my manners? Let me introduce you. This is your body. This is your body on yoga…any questions? I thought there might be, so let's jump in!

We are inhabitants of an amazing and awe-inspiring vehicle. These vehicles allow us to run, jump, dance, shimmy, kiss, hug, read, sing, and learn new things. They allow us to stretch, bend, contort, and stand strong in our yoga postures. Unfortunately, for some reason, we are more likely to study how our new fancy pants smart phone works than the beautiful potential of who we are and what we can do. It is unfortunate, especially because you are likely to only have your phone for a few years, but with care and some luck, you can walk around in these elegant forms for 80-100 years!

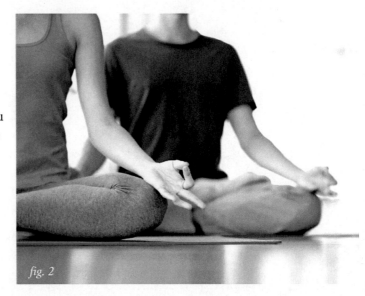

fig. 2

Even in our beloved definition of yoga, there is inspiration to study anatomy. The word yoga is often translated as "union," "to unite," or to "yoke together." Some might say this means to unite with yourself or where you are. Others say it might mean to find union with your higher self or universal consciousness. If you look at the root of the Sanskrit word yoga - yuj - it is from the same root that our English (from the Latin) word jugular comes. The jugular veins in our body connect the head back to the heart; perhaps this can be poetically resonant of the practice that has the ability to unite us back to our heart center

As students and teachers of yoga, it is when we begin to understand the different characters that make up the body that we can then ask them to do what they do best. We can harness our innate power and stop asking for things that are not on our "body resumé" to prevent pain and injury.

Sometimes, studying anatomy can seem overwhelming at first. You can think about it like learning a new language. Once you learn a few key phrases, it becomes easier to understand the language of your form.

Let's begin at the beginning. We have to have a starting point, a home base, and agreed upon neutral before we learn how to safely and efficiently move away from there. In anatomical terms, it's called anatomical position, which looks a whole heck of a lot like our yoga posture Tadasana.

The subject or yogi is standing in front of the observer. Her feet are flat on the floor facing forward and underneath her hips. Her arms are by her side with the palms of her hands facing forward and she is looking straight ahead. From here we can reference different parts or locations by using the following terms:

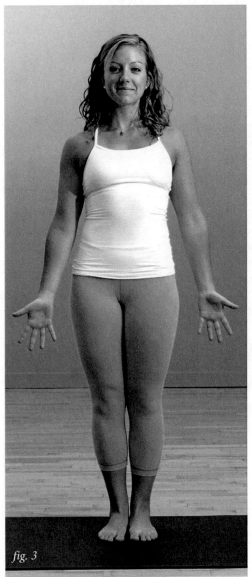

fig. 3

Anterior: near the front of the body; in front of

Posterior: near the back of the body; behind (I remember this like, *"Dude! He's got a nice posterior!"* but that's just me.)

Superior: above

Inferior: below

Lateral: toward the side; away from the midline

Medial: toward the midline

Distal: away from; farther away from the origin

Proximal: near; closer to the origin

Superficial: toward the surface

Deep: closer to the core

Now that we have some direction, let's meet the characters in the body play.

Chapter 2

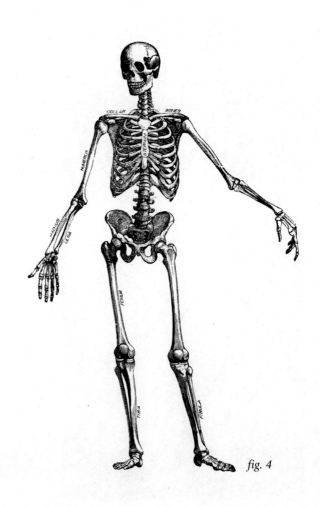

fig. 4

Them Bones, Them bones
THE EXQUISITE SKELETAL STRUCTURE

"To live in this world, you must
be able to do three things:
to love what is mortal; to hold
it against your bones knowing
your life depends on it; and,
when the time comes to let it
go, to let it go."

- MARY OLIVER

There are 206 bones, give or take a few, in your adult body. We say, "give or take a few," because we are actually born with quite a few more - around 300. As we age, some of these bones ossify, or join together. It's also really important to remember that though we study the average body in our anatomy classes, there is a huge variety of human anatomy. For instance, 1 in 20 people will have an extra rib! Ten percent of the population has an extra vertebra! I've been lucky enough to see many bones and skeletons in my life, and I can safely say that no 2 are exactly alike!

While we cannot X-ray our students as they come in to our classrooms and see all of this variety, we must remember that every skeleton is slightly different. Along with muscle, ligament, energy, constitution, and mood, your students are all wildly unique! As teachers, we must remember this and not ask for a "cookie cutter" posture or demand that every student do the postures in the same way. It's just not anatomically possible! For example, depending on where your hip sockets face and how the bones articulate together, it may be impossible to get your knees to the floor in a seated crossed leg posture...and that's ok! If, as teachers, we try to push those knees down or tell your students to "keep working on it and it will come," this could and will lead to injury. While there are some tricks to determine if the restriction is bony (that ain't changing) or muscular (could change), our best bet is to support our students to find the presence inside their posture rather than some idealized shape.

When people ask me what my favorite body system is (full disclosure: not many people really ask me this), I have to say the skeletal system. While admittedly not as sexy as the nervous system, it definitely holds a special place in my heart. It's easy to view the skeleton as just a functional and structural element there to keep us from being amorphous blobs. This unjust view is not helped by the fact that as anatomy students we are often shown plastic models and two-dimensional Halloween drawings of the skeletal form that belies its magnificent truth. The skeleton is living, dynamic, ever changing, and remodeling tissue! In fact, due to this remodeling, you have a completely different skeleton every 7-10 years. Set in the fluid bath of your body it can have the tensile strength of steel but a touch of elasticity like a reed of bamboo: strong, yet yielding.

The skeletal system is made up of different types of cells. Two different cells called osteoblasts and osteoclasts are constantly remodeling the bones. When you think of your muscles leveraging movement, think of trying to lift a bowling ball. Muscles, via their tendons, pull on the outer stocking that's around your bones called the periosteum. With this healthy stress

We are not built the same so posture may vary

WOW↓

applied, the bone underneath (osteoclasts) starts to break down. This sends out a call of, *"Hey! I'm breaking down over here! Let's make more bone cells."* Osteoblasts mobilize to build up bone under that stress. This is the basis on which bones heal after a fracture.

This dance of breaking down and building up of bone tissue begins to wane as we get older. With more breaking down than building up happening, we are sometimes left with small "holes" inside our honeycomb-like bones which leads to lower bone density, weakness in the bones, and possible fractures. This is emphasized in women because of how special hormonal changes act on calcium and can lead to a higher rate of osteoporosis. Often, doctors will prescribe weight-bearing exercise (and, by the way, yoga is a weight-bearing exercise) to help stimulate bone integrity to prepare for their stronger muscles.

A real bone specimen is quite different from its plastic, anatomical model counterpart. The skeleton, like the soft skin on our non-botoxed face, is a road map to every experience that has touched us. It begins to tell the story of our lives to those who have grown quiet and skilled enough to hear it. I always feel a rush of excitement at the notion of something seemingly unyielding and static blossom into something that screams potential! That's what the skeleton feels like to me: a snapshot of your past, but also a vehicle for the ever changing.

When studying the skeleton, we can divide it into two important parts: **the axial skeleton** and **the appendicular skeleton**.

The axial skeleton, just like it sounds, forms the axis of the body. It includes:

Skull (cranium/maxilla): the skull is made up of several different bones, but for our purposes, we will just lump them together

Mandible: jawbone

The Ossicles (Incus/Malleus/Stapes): teeny tiny bones of the inner ear

Hyoid: U-shaped bone in the throat area to which your tongue attaches

Vertebral Column: made up of 24 individual articulating vertebra plus the sacrum and coccyx

Ribs: Twelve pairs of ribs: R1-R7 true ribs, R8-R10 false ribs, R11-R12 floating ribs

Axial Skeleton

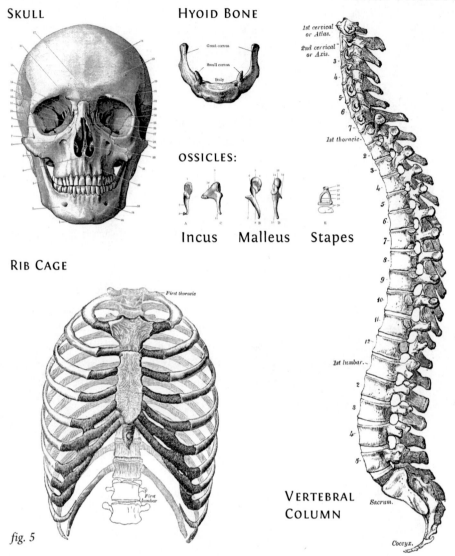

SKULL

HYOID BONE

OSSICLES:

Incus Malleus Stapes

RIB CAGE

fig. 5

VERTEBRAL
COLUMN

The appendicular skeleton, like it sounds, includes the bones of the appendages:

Clavicle: collarbone

Scapula: shoulder blade

Humerus: upper arm bone

Radius: thumb-side forearm bone

Ulna: pinky-side forearm bone

Carpals: Eight pebble-like bones in each wrist area *who knew*

Metacarpals: distal to, or beyond the carpals

Phalanges: fingers

Pelvis: made up of three parts: ilium, ischium, pubis

Femur: upper leg bone; longest bone in the body

Patella: kneecap

Tibia: medial shin bone

Fibula: lateral shin bone

Tarsus: Seven rock-like bones in each foot

Metatarsals: Distal to, or beyond the tarsus

Phalanges: toes

Appendicular Skeleton

SHOULDER GRIDLE

ARM

LEG

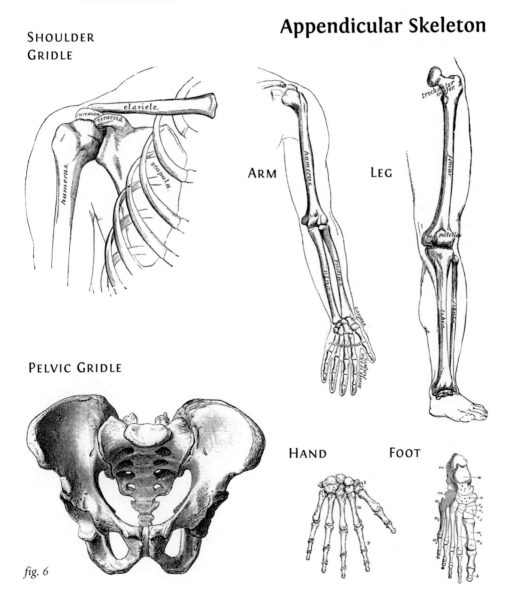

PELVIC GRIDLE

HAND

FOOT

fig. 6

To move our bodies, our muscles pull on these bones and leverage movement across the joints in three planes:

Sagittal plane

Think of a line that could cut you into right and left pieces. This could be right down your very center (midsagittal) or anywhere cutting you into uneven right and left halves. Movements along this plane are called flexion and extension.

Flexion- movement that decreases the angle between the two parts at the joint. Bending your elbow or your knees when you're sitting down are good examples of flexion.

Extension- movement that increases the angle between the two parts at the joint. The back leg in a lunge is in extension at the hip. When your elbows and knees straighten, or when you arch your neck to look up at the moon, they are in extension.

The phrase double jointed usually refers to a joint that moves beyond its normal limits. The prefix hyper- is often added, like hyper-flexion or hyper-extension of these joints. This could be due to how the bones fit together or laxity of the ligaments surrounding and supporting the joint (more on this to come).

Coronal Plane

Think of a line that could cut you into anterior (front) and posterior (back) pieces. The movements that are available in this plane are abduction and adduction.

Abduction- Away from the midline. Think of aliens abducting you. Yes, that's what I said. They would take you away from your home; away from the midline. Your arms in Warrior 2 and your legs in a wide leg forward bend are in abduction.

Adduction- Toward the midline. Think of adding two numbers together. Adduction is a movement that pulls a structure back toward the midline or across the midline. Dropping the arms in Warrior 2 or eagle legs are in adduction.

Transverse Plane

Think of a line that would cut you into superior (top) and inferior (bottom) pieces. This could be right in the center or anywhere cutting you into uneven top and bottom pieces. Movements that are available in this plane are called rotation. Rotation in the spine is usually just referred to as rotating right or left.

External Rotation (lateral rotation) - Turning your legs (femurs) out like a dancer might or rolling the arm bones (humerus) open in downward facing dog are good examples of external rotation.

Internal Rotation (medial rotation) - Rotating the arms or legs inward so the toes or flexed forearm would point towards the midline. The opposite of external rotation.

Ok, that might have been a whole bunch of new words. If you're feeling overwhelmed, get up, take a deep breath, go stretch your legs, and then meet me at the coolest joint in town.

Chapter 3

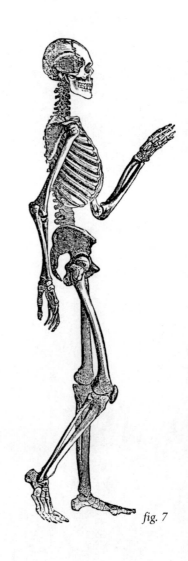

fig. 7

Do You Come To This Joint Often?

THE CHARACTERS IN A SYNOVIAL JOINT

" "The body is shaped, disciplined, honored, and in time, trusted"

- MARTHA GRAHAM

Bones articulate together to form a joint. There are many different types of joints. For example, all the bones of the skull (except the mandible) are joined together by sutures, a type of synarthrotic (immoveable) joints. Your teeth articulate with your mandible and maxilla with a joint called a gomphosis, another type of synarthrotic joint. While these are certainly cool to discuss, I rarely find myself instructing students to try to move their left incisor medially or try to align their skull plates. So, we will stick mostly to what are called diarthrotic, or freely moveable synovial joints.

Many factors will contribute to the amount of range of motion (ROM) available in a joint. The way the bones articulate with one another, the structural and functional classification of the joint, as well as the laxity of the ligaments and muscles in the region all help determine what a joint is able to do. This is highly individual and yet another reason we can't expect the same range from each student. As my teacher Alan Finger is fond of saying, *"Range is of the ego; form is of the soul."*

Although sometimes the names will be slightly different, all synovial joints will have a lot of the same characteristics. First, there is an articulation between two or more bones. Surrounding this articulation will be a joint capsule, a fibrous membrane which encapsulates the joint. Its inner membrane, the synovial membrane, will produce a fluid which, by no surprise, is called synovial fluid. The synovial fluid is a clear lubricating fluid that reduces heat and friction as the joint moves. It also acts as a nutrient and oxygen transport and helps to remove waste products and carbon dioxide. It contains a type of cell that eats up the debris inside the joint, helping to keep the joint tidy.

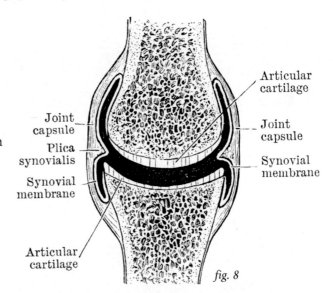

Joint capsule
Plica synovialis
Synovial membrane
Articular cartilage
Articular cartilage
Joint capsule
Synovial membrane

fig. 8

You've most likely heard some noises coming from your body. Well, let me be more specific here. You may have heard a snap, crackle, and pop sound coming from your joints as you move around. Typically, this is not dangerous.

It's usually just gas bubbles popping inside the joint capsule. Some people are just gassier than others. Think of a closed water bottle. Like the joint capsule, it's an enclosed space filled with fluid. If you were to shake your water bottle, you would observe bubbles forming and popping. This will often happen in the normal movement of your joints. Of course, if you are always popping in one specific joint or movement, or if it causes pain, it's worth further investigation. At this point, you might be thinking of that old piece of folksy wisdom from Grandma: "*If you keep cracking your knuckles like that, you are going to get arthritis!*" Short answer is: Grandma is wrong (sorry Nana). The more complicated answer is: she is sort of right. Usually, when you see someone "go for a crack," he or she is aggressively and habitually manipulating the joints in a way that they actually don't anatomically move. This could very well lead us down a path to osteoarthritis, which we will explain more as we get deeper into these joints.

Now, we have to have a support structure that keeps these articulating bones aligned; this is the job of the ligaments. Ligaments are bands of connective tissue that passively reinforce the joints to prevent undesirable movement. While they have a little bit of give, they are not very elastic, and if overstretched, will never return to their cute spring-chicken length. They are also virtually avascular, meaning they have no direct blood supply to transport new nutrients and proteins to help rebuild and repair damage. Because of this, if you injure a ligament, healing is very troublesome. If the ligaments are put offline due to over stretching or injury, this allows the two articulating bones to rub in an inappropriate way (get your minds out of the gutter), and can easily lead to damage to some of the structures inside the joint.

In some joints like the shoulder, hip, knee, and in between the vertebra you will find a special type of cartilage called fibrocartilage. This fibrocartilage will have special names like labrums, meniscus, and discs depending on their location, but all will act as shock absorbers. They hold space in the joint, help to deepen the congruency and provide a more snuggly fit between the two articulating bones. Think of your head hitting your pillow at the end of the night; as it snuggles down into the cushioning of the pillow, more surface area of your head touches your pillow's surface. Much like the ligaments, these dense pieces of connective tissue are avascular and will be tough or near impossible to heal.

Painted on the ends of the articular surfaces of the bones is something called articular or hyaline cartilage. I always think of it like nail polish painted onto the ends of the bones. It's a glassy, smooth, and shiny cartilage

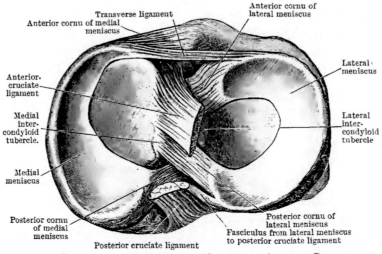

PROXIMAL END OF TIBIA WITH MENISCI AND ATTACHED PORTIONS OF CRUCIATE LIGAMENTS.

fig. 9

that provides one last layer of shock absorption and prevents the bones from rubbing against one another. Just like nail polish, it can get chipped, and will not regenerate due to it being avascular as well.

Yoga postures can be a brilliant tonic to help support and nourish joint health but unfortunately can also, if not careful, cause a lot of trouble to these structures. For example, a lot of our postures call for external rotation of the hip and flexion of the knee (pigeon, ankle to knee, cobblers pose, lotus, etc.). When we reach the limit of our range of motion in the hip but still try to move deeper into the pose, the stress will often move into the knee. As the knee tries to compensate and give you some rotation (not really on its joint resumé) the result is often an over stretching of the ligaments. Then the bones will rub and grate on the meniscus, possibly wearing it down enough to start chipping the articular cartilage, thus exposing the bone to stress. As we remember from our last chapter, the reaction of this stress on the bone will start to break down the bone, in turn sending the call out for more bone to run to the area. This often causes little bony stalagmites and stalactites (osteophytes) to form inside the joint, limiting the mobility, and causing a lot of pain and swelling. These little bony outgrowths can also break off and float around in the joint, something doctors coyly name joint mice. While this visual may be cute, the osteoarthritis process is most definitely not. Yet another reason for us to work on finding the presence inside the posture rather than trying to always get deeper or more out of a posture.

In your body's high traffic zones where a lot of different tissues are running over each other, you will often find structures called bursa. Bursa are

Attempting to dupen unto a yose can cause osteoarthritis

synovial fluid filled sacs akin to a soft squishy marble that help provide more cushioning and a slip-and-slide between body tissues. Just like most things in the body, they can get aggravated. Often, when there is an inflammation to a tissue, the suffix -itis is added. A bursitis (inflammation to the bursa) will result when there is a rubbing or irritation of the bursa.

Surrounding the joint you have your highly vascular and super cool skeletal muscles. Skeletal muscles have very different properties than the structures that we have named above.

They have **excitability**, or the ability to receive and respond to stimuli.

They have **contractility**, or the ability to contract forcibly when stimulated.

They have **extensibility**, or the ability to be stretched.

They have **elasticity**, or the ability to recoil back to their resting length after being stretched.

If you have eaten meat (apologies to my fellow vegetarians), what you are eating are the animal's muscles. From afar, it just looks like a hunk of meat, but as you look closer, you can notice that it is a bunch of smaller fibers. If you could look even closer, you would notice that each of these fibers are actually made up of even smaller fibers. Each small fiber is made up of proteins. Filaments slide past one another like inchworms producing a contraction that changes both the length and shape of the cell. Each level of organization of fibers is covered in a sheath of fascia. Fascia is like your body's Saran Wrap, and encases every muscle, nerve and organ. The outreach of your muscles' fascia extends to form tough fibrous bands of tissue called tendons. Tendons will attach muscle to bone by knitting into the periosteum, or outer stocking. Tendons will help to transmit the force of a muscle, help to stabilize a joint, and may in some cases act as a spring to help in efficiency of some movements.

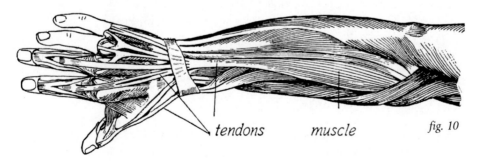

tendons   *muscle*   *fig. 10*

Muscles are innervated by your nerves. When your muscle receives the signal from your nerves to contract, it pulls one bone of a joint towards the other, leveraging the movement. Muscles work in pairs and teams to help facilitate movement at your joints.

Stretching likes to happen in the belly of the muscle. The fascia, tendons, and ligaments will follow the lead of the muscles. There are safety measures imbedded in the nerves of the muscles and tendons that will ultimately try to control the limits of the stretch. They send out pain and spasm signals to warn us when we are in danger of going too far and injuring those tissues.

A muscle can contract in a few different ways:

It can **concentrically contract**, or shorten as it contracts, like your bicep muscle as you try to lift your bowling ball.

It can **eccentrically contract**, or lengthen as it contacts, like your bicep slowly lowering the bowling ball once you've picked it up.

It can **statically contract**, like when after picking up your bowling ball, you freeze and realize that you don't even know how to bowl and you're not really sure what to do with it. The biceps would be working (isometrically), but the muscle would be neither lengthening nor shortening.

Muscles will also play different roles:

Agonists or prime movers are the main muscle for the job. They do the job or action most efficiently.

Synergists are the helper muscles which fine tune and support the prime mover in its action.

Antagonists are muscles usually on the opposite side of the joint to the prime mover. Just like the antagonist in a movie, they oppose the action of the hero of the story, or the agonists. They often help to monitor, smooth, and slow the movement to protect the joint.

Stabilizers are muscles that will work in opposition to each other to maintain a bone in place.

As we have all experienced in asana, it's wonderfully complicated as many different actions occur across many different joints using many different muscles doing many different jobs.

Chapter 4

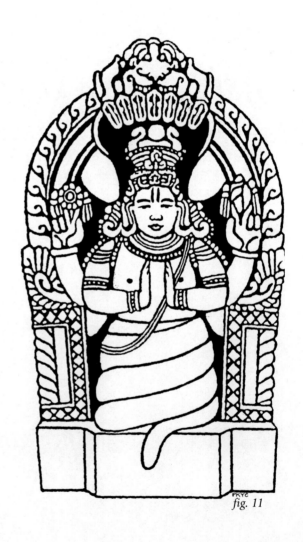

fig. 11

We Interrupt This Book With a Message From Patanjali

YOGA SUTRAS BREAK

"For those who have an intense urge for Spirit and wisdom, it sits near them, waiting"

- PATANJALI

In not only the physical science, but in the real mental silence, the wisdom dawns.

- SWAMI SATCHIDANANDA, THE YOGA SUTRAS

Now is a good time to slow down and remember the beautiful context in which this practice is set. There is a very old text that a lot of yoga teachers like to talk about called, The Yoga Sutras of Patanjali. Although yoga scholars will frequently debate about the author, his lineage, and the time in which the text was written, it serves as an excellent foundation, laying out the philosophy on which this practice stands. Even though the Sutras are said to have been written anywhere from 100 BCE-500 CE, it is resonant to modern yogis on both an esoteric and physical level.

The word sutra often gets translated as "thread" or "aphorism". There are 195 small threads or statements that sometimes seem intentionally vague or difficult; I believe it's to encourage thoughtful contemplation and discussion with a guide, teacher, or fellow student. The word suture, as in when a doctor sutures a wound together, comes from the same root as sutra, which may hint to this book helping to stitch together the fracture or wound between spirit/self or self/others.

While all the sutras are relevant to us as we move through this practice, I'd like to talk about the 3 that have really made a difference in my asana and teaching.

1:1 Atha Yoga Anusasanam

The Yoga Sutras of Patanjali is divided into four chapters, or padas. This sutra is the very first line in the first chapter entitled Samadhi Pada (chapter on equal reflection or enlightenment). Patanjali doesn't pull any punches. He starts off big with describing the state of total absorption. Some have said this bold move was to inspire students on this path, others suggest it was assuming the student has already had some experience and wanted to understand the experience or put it into context. Many different scholars will debate about the meaning and translation of these sutras. Even more challenging, they are written in Sanskrit - notoriously hard to translate as each word has several different interpretations. Most teachers seem to agree on the first word: Atha. Atha is defined as "now" and it seems telling that this book begins with this exclamation rather than "once upon a time" or "someday in your future." Some say this sutra translates as, "now the exposition or teaching of Yoga is being made," perhaps meaning that there is a direct practice being illuminated rather than an esoteric philosophy. Others state that using the word "now" indicates that there was a "before," and that the teachings, teachers, and preparation had been underway before the sutras. My favorite interpretation is my current teacher's translation: "Yoga (or union) can only occur in the moment of now."

Training the mind to move back to the here and now is a challenge. We have programmed our minds to project where we would like to go and what we would like to achieve as well as to peruse and marinate in the past. Rarely do we allow ourselves to come fully congruent with where we are. Often when there is a pause in our day or in our minds we quickly look to fill it with a conversation, email, text, Facebook, Instagram, Pinterest...well, you get my point. The more we allow ourselves to move back into the place where we are, in this moment of now, without immediately trying to distract or change it, the more we begin to notice the transient nature of the mind, emotions, and beliefs. This remembrance makes it less tempting to try to attach to or push away any of these things because you know they will not last. Better yet, it's far less tempting to identify any of that as who you are.

Coming back to the "now" in our asana practice allows us to identify more with what is actually occurring in our bodies and minds and less with trying to achieve a certain aesthetic or reminiscing about how you used to feel in a posture. This lets us connect in a way that is ultimately safer for our physical bodies and more peaceful and quieting to our minds. As we train our minds to return back into this moment of "now," we can experience this greater connection to the state beyond the mind, connection to our higher self, or to the unified field of energy (really, the state beyond name and form).

Being present in our practice

2:1 Tapah Svadhyayesvara Pranidhanani Kriya Yogah

Ok, that's a lot of large words, so let's take them one by one. This sutra *rule.* is the very first line in the second chapter entitled Sadhana Pada. Sadhana Pada, or the portion on practice, begins to share how to find this state of connection or bliss. Tapah or Tapas in this context are not the yummy treats you get in your neighborhood Spanish restaurant, but rather translates as, "to burn, austerity or discipline." Isvara pranidhanam (slightly different transliteration when taken out of the sutra) means, "surrender, softening, to give over or release." The word in the middle of these two is Svadhyaya, meaning the "study of the sva or self." Rounding out the sutra, the two words Kriya yogah mean "the action or practice of this yoga (union)."

The practice of finding this union that we seek is found by the balance of discipline and surrender. The only way we know how much of each of these we need to create this balance is by the watchful study of ourselves. Much like a beginner tightrope walker, at first we are pretty unstable at this delicate dance and fall in one direction or the other. As we keep studying ourselves, with practice, we are able to walk through more gracefully. Even the most skillful tightrope walker will always maintain a slight negotiation from side to side to keep his or her balance.

In our physical asana practice, it becomes important to learn how to have both discipline and surrender. We need discipline to have a consistent practice and also to engage with where we are. There is even discipline needed to energize a pose so you don't hang into the joints, possibly causing injury. Of course, this discipline needs to be balanced with soft surrender in order to come back into the presence inside the posture rather than trying to work the pose harder. It's a fine line that we walk here, and only by checking in and observing ourselves do we walk it with comfort and ease.

2:46 Sthira Sukham Asanam

A little bit later on in the Sadhana Pada lies this lovely jewel. Some yogis say that this particular sutra is the only one that directly relates to how our asana posture practice should be performed. I disagree. I see every aspect of this philosophy as both a tool for the mind but also in the physical structures of the body.

The word Sthira is translated as, "structure, steadiness, support, or boundaries." Sukham is a beautiful word meaning, "good space" or "sweetness" (like the French word sucre). While asanam is often translated to mean the postures we do in our yoga classes, more specifically, and I think intentionally, it means "seat." I think the use of the word "seat" also opens this up to how we sit in all relationships. Whether with our bodies, our down dog, or a loved one, our relationships should have the qualities of spaciousness, sweetness, and openness, but with boundaries and structure. One without the other creates imbalance. Because this is not a book on love relationships (unless you count my great love of the bones), we will stick to the physical form here.

Everything likes to have its own "good space" in the body, and the joints are no exception. It's like when there are too many people in a subway car; at first you can handle it, but as more and more people get on the train, even the most yogic amongst us can't help but get aggravated. We can learn in this physical practice to hold space or sukham in the joints while using the muscular body scaffolding to support and create boundaries. It's important to remember in a practice that seems to celebrate openness, stretching further, and going deeper, that the opposing qualities of strength and boundaries are equally of value for the health and longevity of the physical form.

Chapter 5

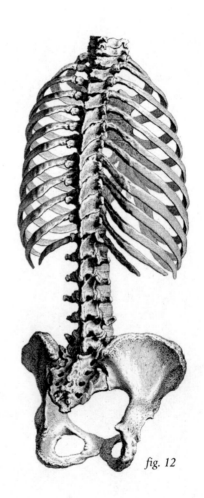

fig. 12

I've Got Your Back, Jack!

THE GLORY OF THE SPINE

> "Much of man's character will be found betokened in his backbone. I would rather feel your spine than your skull, whoever you are..."
>
> - HERMAN MELVILLE

The stunning architecture of the spine plays an extremely important role in our bodies. It supports and distributes the weight of the upper form, provides posture, and allows for movement, all while protecting the graceful tissues of the spinal cord. Its curvy nature evolved to help us leverage the limbs, giving us the unique distinction as bipedal mammals (fancy-pants name for upright critters). While we are often asked by our moms or yoga teachers to "straighten our spines," we have these elegant and meaningful curves for a reason, and they should be supported and maintained whenever possible.

There are 24 individual articulating vertebrae as well as the fused bones of the sacrum and coccyx which make up this great column. These bones can be separated into different regions and curves. While most vertebrae have a similar structure, each region of the spine has slight anomalies - enough to make big differences to the type of movement allowed in each region.

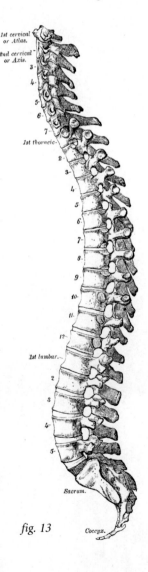

7 cervical vertebrae (C1-C7)

12 thoracic vertebrae (T1-T12)

5 lumbar vertebrae (L1-L5)

4-5 fused sacral vertebrae (S1-S5)

3-5 fused coccygeal vertebrae
Coc 1- Coc 4)

In the adult spine, we can acknowledge four distinct curves:

Cervical - lordotic or concave

Thoracic- kyphotic or convex

Lumbar - lordotic or concave

Sacral/coccygeal - kyphotic or convex

fig. 13

On the streets, in anatomy slang, you might hear something like, *"Dude, she's really lordotic!"* meaning she has an exaggerated lumbar curve. Or perhaps, *"Wow! He's really kyphotic!"* meaning the fella has an exaggerated thoracic curve. The reality is that we adults all have two kyphotic curves and two lordotic curves, even though sometimes the term loosely refers to the exaggeration. The lateral and rotational deviation of the spine is called scoliosis. Those with scoliosis have very unique anatomy which will take much more individual study to address in a yoga practice.

If you have a baby, or have ever seen a baby, you've probably noticed that they look a little like a shrimp when they come out. Cute, adorable shrimp, but shrimp nonetheless. They are born with only the primary curves of the thoracic and sacral/coccygeal, giving them this comma-like shape. This is why you are (hopefully) told to not try to sit them up or hold them without supporting their little heads and necks because they will just flop back into this shape, not being able to hold the position. As this adorable floppy baby grows, she is probably given something called "tummy time." This is when her parents put her on her belly and in an attempt to see what's going on around her, she has to work her cervical muscles, developing her cervical curve. A little later, she will begin to push herself up on to her hands and knees in what will look like a baby cat and cow pose. She will also start to throw herself back, terrifying anyone who is holding her, and pull herself back up. This is like little baby crunches working her abdominals, all in an effort to develop the lumbar curve. Now that she has the secondary lordotic curves of the cervical and lumbar, she can now begin to pull herself up to stand and take those first wobbly steps. Ah, they grow up so fast, don't they?

The lumbar curve is unique to humans and allows us to have the leverage, shock absorption, and balance to ambulate on our feet. You might have seen trained chimps taught to walk upright in an effort to look more human. If you've noticed, they throw their long arms overhead and slightly behind them to create a mock lumbar curve, allowing them to temporarily walk upright.

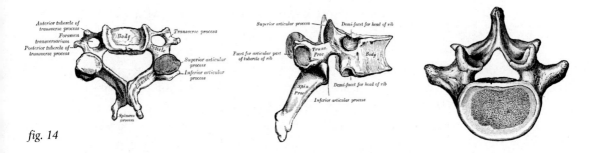

fig. 14

Most individual vertebra will have a similar appearance. Anteriorly, they have a vertebral body that supports and translates much of the weight. Posteriorly, they have a beak like projection called a spinous process and two lateral projections called transverse processes. Anything that's pointy on a bone, like these processes, is a great place for muscle and ligament attachment. These three projections create a vertebral arch and the negative space is called the vertebral foramen. When you line up all of the vertebral foramen, you have the vertebral canal in which the spinal cord descends. Where the vertebral arch meets the body of the vertebra, you have two small facets. Most vertebrae will articulate with their neighbors at three joints: the two facets and the vertebral bodies. They rest upon each other like a milking stool, and when properly aligned, provide strength and stability in the column.

In between all but the first two vertebrae rests a special piece of fibrocartilage called the intervertebral disc. This disc is often compared to a stale jelly doughnut. It has a tough fibrous shell called the annulus fibrosus and a jelly-like center called the nucleus pulposus. These "doughnuts" help to distribute the weight in the intervertebral joint and act as shock absorbers. If you imagine pressing down on the front or anterior of the

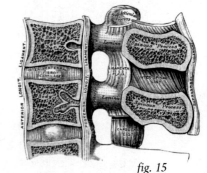

fig. 15

jelly doughnut, like in flexion of the spine, the jelly will be smushed posteriorly. Pressing down on the posterior, as in extension of the spine, the jelly will be smushed anteriorly. When we twist or rotate our spine, the two bodies of the vertebra will move closer together, and the jelly will be squashed in all directions.

The way the discs maintain their health and plumpness is through movement. When you move the spine, the discs will get wrung out like a dirty sponge, and when you release the movement, the discs will drink from the neighboring tissues. You might have heard that if you were to measure yourself first thing in the morning you would be a wee bit taller than if you were to measure yourself before going to bed. This is because of the pull of gravity on our upright bodies compresses the discs, and they lose some of their moisture to the surrounding tissues. As we rest, changing the way gravity affects us, the discs get to plump back up. As we age, though, the discs lose much of their own water content and direct blood supply, leaving them more prone to damage and strain. Weakening or tearing in the outer shell of the disc can allow the jelly to poke its gelatinous head out, otherwise known as a bulging disc. In fact, it's estimated that 60-70% of people over

35 years old will have some kind of deterioration, bulging, or herniated disc (this is where the jelly spurts out). The good news is: depending on the direction in which it pokes its head, you could be completely asymptomatic. Unfortunately, most of the time, the jelly will begin to protrude laterally and posteriorly. This puts it at risk of pressing into the spinal cord or spinal nerve roots, causing pain, tingling, or numbness along the path which that particular nerve travels. Without surgical intervention, the jelly will never snuggle neatly back into the doughnut and will always be compromised. Much of the work in physical and yoga therapy is to create more space between the affected vertebrae and to shore them up with the surrounding muscles to help hold that space. Observing postural imbalance is also key to help lessen the chance for the disc to irritate the nerves again. While the possibility of injury in all regions of the spine exists because of the weight supported, amount of movement and postural pitfalls, the lumbar region wins as the most prone to these disc injuries.

Each region of the spine is unique. The mobility of each vertebra is determined by its bony projections, its surroundings, and how things fit together. Let's take a look at one section at a time, but keep in mind that most complex yoga movements involving the spine involve many vertebrae across many regions.

Cervical Vertebrae

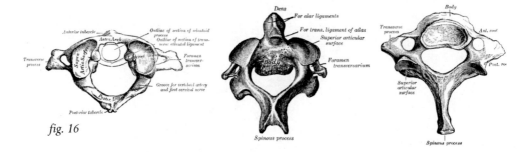

fig. 16

There are seven cervical vertebrae making up the lordotic cervical curve. C1 and C2 are unique and have been given their own special names: the atlas and the axis. The atlas, named after the Greek Titan who held up the celestial sphere, articulates with the base of the skull. It is a big bony ring with no vertebral body or processes. It sits upon C2, or the axis, which has a superiorly projecting phallus called the dens. This allows the skull and C1 to pivot as if you were saying no. C3-C7 have small vertebral bodies designed by evolution to support the fairly light weight of the head. C7 is unique in that it has a long and prominent spinous process which can usually be seen or felt on the base of your neck. Most of the cervical spine's flexion and extension takes place at the alanto-occipital joint (where your skull meets C1), but is aided by the other vertebrae in this region. Most of the rotation available in the cervical region will take place in the atlanto-axial joint (C1/C2), but, like in all movements, is usually facilitated by multiple joints.

In the transverse process of every cervical vertebra you will find small foramina (holes) in which the special vertebral arteries will rise. These are fountains of oxygen-rich blood that feed the brain. Housed in a delicate bony ring, they are not usually put in jeopardy, but in yoga we have the audacity to stand on our heads and do other wildly funky things with our necks. The small vertebral bodies are poorly equipped to support the weight of the entire body like we ask of them in headstand. Yogis will often try to throw their heads back in extreme extension or rotate the neck beyond the limits in certain poses, which is a dangerous combination of rotation and extension. All of these actions put the intervertebral discs and vertebral arteries at risk for injury. This doesn't mean that healthy individuals can't do these postures, but they must employ other intelligence because the structure is not well suited for it. Proper and conservative alignment for the head and neck must be maintained to keep this mobile and dainty area safe.

Thoracic Vertebrae

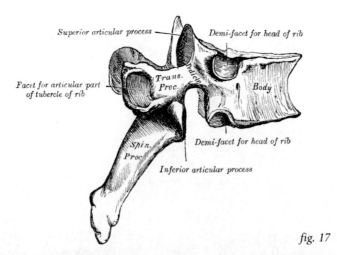

fig. 17

There are 12 thoracic vertebrae making up the kyphotic thoracic curve. They are intermediate in size, and as the heart shaped vertebral bodies descend, they get slightly larger to support the increasing weight from the upper form and extremity. The spinous processes in this region project sharply inferior and each vertebra will articulate with a pair of ribs. This greatly limits the amount of movement allowed in each joint. Most movement will come from a combination of vertebrae rather than just one vertebral joint. Extension will be limited by the toucan beak-like spinous processes and individual flexion; rotation and side bending (lateral flexion) will be limited by the ribs.

You have 12 pairs of ribs articulating with the 12 thoracic vertebrae. Ribs 1-7 (true ribs) articulate directly with the sternum anteriorly via its own road of cartilage called the costal cartilage. Ribs 8-10 (false ribs) articulate via a multilane costal cartilage highway that merges into one attachment at the sternum. This will make a slight difference in mobility to the vertebrae to which they are attached. T11 and T12 articulate with Ribs 11 and 12 (floating ribs). These ribs don't reach around to attach to the sternum and can be felt easily on the side, waist, and back. Because there are no connections of these ribs to the sternum anteriorly, these vertebrae will have much more range compared to their other thoracic brethren.

Lumbar Vertebrae

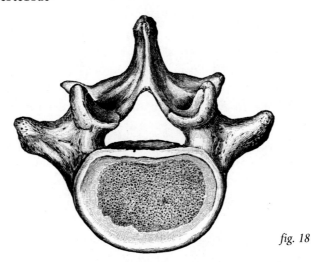

fig. 18

There are 5 lumbar vertebrae making up the lordotic lumbar curve. They have large vertebral bodies that are well suited to support weight. Having robust, stout spinous processes that don't run into each other quickly means flexion and extension are readily available. The transverse processes are fairly rectangular and project laterally, preventing a great amount of lateral flexion (side bending) and rotation. Because of the large range of flexion and extension, the large weight they support, and the shearing movement of these vertebrae, the articulation between the lower lumbar vertebrae and the lumbar-sacral joint is a site of frequent injury.

Sacrum

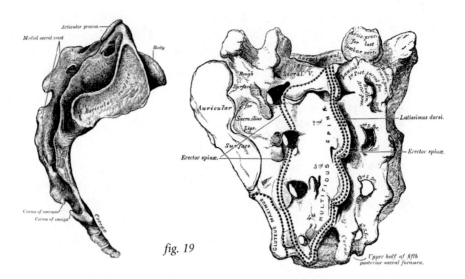

fig. 19

The sacrum is a pyramid-shaped bone with its apex pointing downward. It is said to be made up of 4-5 fused vertebrae. The sacrum and tailbone are curved convexly, contributing to this kyphotic curve. Out of all the bones that I've seen, the sacrum has the most variety. Size, shape, articulation, and number of vertebrae all vary from person to person, making a huge difference in mobility and stability of the surrounding joints.

Superiorly, the sacrum articulates with the fifth lumbar vertebra. In some cases, an individual can have an extra lumbar vertebra and one less sacral vertebra. This is usually because the first vertebra of the sacrum is not fully fused. This is called lumbarization of the sacrum. In some cases, an individual can have an extra sacral vertebra and one less lumbar vertebra, called sacralization of the lumbar region.

Laterally, the sacrum articulates with the ilia (part of the pelvis) at the sacroiliac joints (SI joints). There is some debate as to whether the sacrum has independent movement from the ilia, or if the sacrum just goes along for the ride as the pelvic bowl moves. Any independent movement allowed in this joint is limited as this joint is the fulcrum between the upper body and the legs and is meant to be quite strong and stable. The sacrum, moving along with the pelvic bowl, can be thought of as nodding or nutating. As you tip the pelvic bowl forward, as if you are spilling its contents anteriorly, the top of the sacrum moves anteriorly or nutates. As you tip the pelvic bowl backwards, as if you are spilling its contents posteriorly, the top of the sacrum moves posteriorly or counter-nutates. By opposing these actions often, we bring strain and compression into this area, which can cause a lot dysfunction into this joint. (More about this in the next chapter.)

Due to some differences between the male and female pelvis, the male and female sacrum also differ greatly. The male sacrum is taller and narrower, and articulates at 3 segments with the ilia. The female sacrum is wider and squatter and articulates at only 2 segments. This allows for more potential movement, and thus potential injury, in women's SI joint.

The inferior aspect of the sacrum articulates with the tailbone, or coccyx.

Coccyx

The word coccyx comes from a Greek word meaning cuckoo. This refers to the curved shaped of a cuckoo's beak when viewed from the side. The coccyx is considered to be 3-5 fused vertebrae that articulate with the inferior aspect of the sacrum. There are many anatomy texts that will disagree and classify this joint as either synovial (some movement), fibrocartilaginous (very little movement) or ossified (no movement). While there is a disc in between the sacrum and coccyx, any movement is extremely limited. The coccyx serves as an important attachment site for ligaments, many muscles of the pelvic floor and backside, and the sheaths covering the spinal cord (filum terminale).

To move this column of bones, we need some muscles. Let's begin to look at some of the muscles in the trunk that contribute to the support and movement in this region.

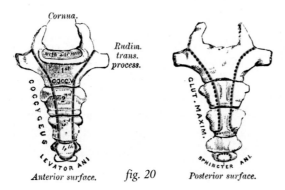

Anterior surface.   *fig. 20*   *Posterior surface.*

Erector Spinae

The erector spinae muscles are actually a large group of deep back muscles that run the length of either side of the spine like railroad tracks. Fibers of these muscles extend from the occiput (base of the skull) to the sacrum and ilia with attachments to the ribs and each vertebra. Just like the name indicates, they help to hold or support the spine erect. When we bilaterally contract them, they take the spine into extension like in our backend salabhasana, or locust pose. We can stretch them by doing forward flexion of the spine like in our cat pose. Because this is such a long group of muscles, it is quite possible to have one area very hypertonic (tight) and another area hypotonic (weak or underutilized). A typical postural pitfall that I see is the pelvis tucked under (posterior tilt) the lumbar and thoracic spine kyphotic. Now because you have to see your computer screen, or where you are going, the neck will hyper extend and the chin will jut forward. This causes the erector spinae fibers in the neck to tighten, and the thoracolumbar fibers to weaken.

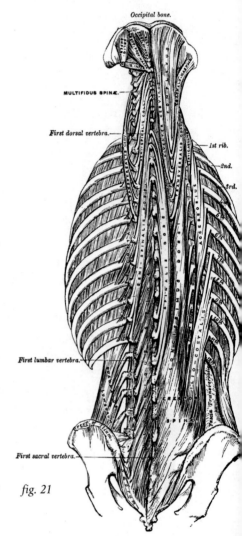

fig. 21

Quadratus Lumborum

The quadratus lumborum is a four-sided rectangular muscle in the lumbar region. It attaches to the posterior side of the ilia, the 12th rib, and the transverse processes of L1-L5. When contracted bilaterally, it helps to extend the lumbar spine, and when contracted unilaterally, it will laterally flex the spine or hike the hip upward. If the pelvis is held in place, contraction of the quadratus lumborum will draw the 12th rib down, aiding in respiration. We can stretch this muscle by flexing the lumbar spine as in cat posture or child's pose. By laterally flexing the spine, we will stretch the quadratus lumborum on the opposite side.

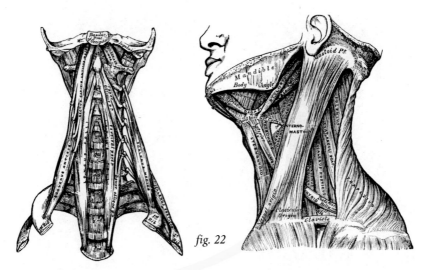

fig. 22

Scalenes

The three scalene muscles run diagonally upward from the top two ribs anteriorly to the transverse processes of the cervical spine. Bilateral contraction will produce flexion of the cervical spine. Working unilaterally as a group, the three scalenes laterally flex the cervical spine. When the cervical spine is fixed, the scalenes' contraction can elevate the first 2 ribs to assist in inhalation.

Sternocleidomastoid

This tongue twister group of muscles is sometimes just referred to as the SCM, and refers to the prominent and visible strap-like muscles in the neck. Originating from both the sternum and the clavicle, they attach to the mastoid process (bumps on your skull that you can feel behind the bottom of your ears). When contracted bilaterally, they help to flex the cervical spine. Contraction unilaterally will create both lateral flexion and rotation to the opposite side in the cervical spine. When the cervical spine is fixed, the SCM helps to lift the sternum and clavicles for greater inspiration.

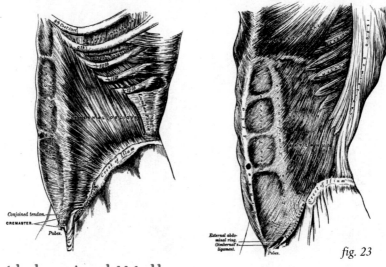

fig. 23

Abdominal Wall

The abdominal wall seen mostly on the anterior of the body is actually a set of 4 muscles that we will name from deepest to most superficial. While each muscle will have distinct actions, in yoga we often try to maintain a light contraction of this muscle group to provide an "air bag" effect. Providing tone in these muscles will protect and support the lumbar curve and help to prevent injury and strain.

Transverse abdominals

The transverse abdominals are the deepest layer of abdominal muscles. Their fibers run in a horizontal pattern forming a deep internal girdle. The fibers have attachments to the thoracolumbar fascia, iliac crest, and lumbar spine on the posterior side, and to the inguinal ligament, ribs 7-12, and linea alba on the anterior side. The linea alba, unlike Jessica Alba, is a tough, fibrous band of tissue that stretches from the xiphoid process to the pubic symphysis. You can place your hands on your belly and cough, belly laugh, or try the breathing technique of Kapalabhati (skull shining breath) and get a sense of this deep internal contraction. I'm going to ask you not to do this now, but the contraction of this muscle will also aid in the act of defecation.

Internal Obliques

These muscles direct diagonally upward and medially toward the linea alba. They attach to the fascia of the lower spine, iliac crest, inguinal ligament, lower ribs, and the linea alba. The internal obliques can be seen as extensions of the internal intercostals (muscles on the internal side of the ribs) which, when contracted, aid in the act of exhalation. When we contract the internal obliques bilaterally, we find flexion of the lower spine. Contraction unilaterally will produce lateral flexion or rotation to the same side.

External Obliques

The external obliques direct diagonally downward and medially towards the linea alba. They have attachments to the lower 8 ribs, illiac crest, and linea alba. They can be seen as extensions of the external intercostals (found on the external surface of the ribs) which, when they contract, aid in inhalation. Contracting the external obliques bilaterally will produce flexion of the lower spine. Unilateral contraction will produce lateral flexion and rotation to the opposite side.

Rectus Abdominals

The rectus abdominals are usually what people think of as the "6-pack" muscles. Due to their superficial nature and the fibrous bands separating the bellies of this muscle, they have a unique and well-known appearance. Actually, in a well defined individual, you might be able to observe an "8-pack" because the linea alba and 4 horizontal fibrous bands create 8 bellies of this muscle. These two parallel muscles run vertically from the pubic crest to the xyphoid process and the cartilage of the fifth, sixth, and seventh ribs. Contraction will produce flexion of the spine.

Chapter 6

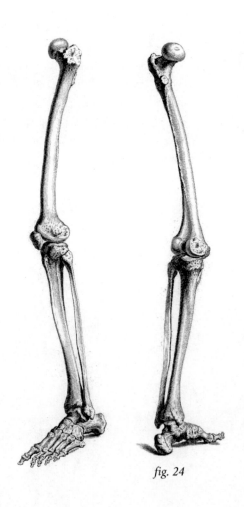

fig. 24

Shake a Leg
ANATOMY OF THE LOWER LIMB

"
"She's got legs, and she knows how to use them"

- ZZ TOP

"

So, how does that song go? The hip bone's connected to the thigh bone... Well that's a good start, but let's look a little closer at this amazing system of ambulation.

Pelvis

The pelvis, derived from the Latin word for basin, can be thought of as a bony bowl. This bowl can be considered as two halves, each half made up of 3 fused bones. Superiorly, we have the ilium. The ilium has special reference points called the iliac crest and the anterior superior iliac spine (ASIS). The iliac crest can be felt, and often seen, as the bony, heart-shaped ridge on the top and sides of our hips. The ASIS are the prominent bony points at the front of our hips often referred to as the hip points. On the posterior and inferior side of this bowl, we find the ischium. The bony protuberances under your butt that you can feel as you wiggle in your chair are your ischial tuberosities, often referred to as your "sitting bones" or "sits bones." This

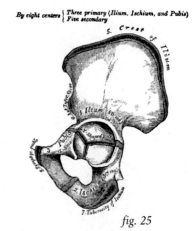

fig. 25

is a little unfortunate because the balance of the pelvis is more complicated than sitting on just your "sitting bones." Tuber comes from the Latin word meaning, "swelling," but we can also think of the ischial tuberosities like tuberous root vegetables. This is why I like to refer to them as the potatoes of the butt. On the anterior side of the pelvis, you will find the pubic bones. The two pubic bones articulate together in the front at the pubic symphysis, a cartilaginous joint. Between the ischial tuberosities and the pubic symphysis, there is a bony bridge contributing to what's called the sub-pubic angle or arch. Each of the three bones that make up the pelvis contributes to the acetabulum, or hip socket.

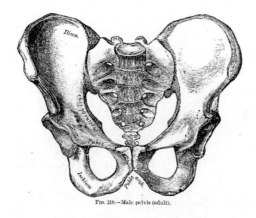

FIG. 210.—Male pelvis (adult).

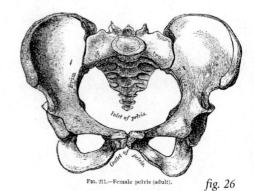

FIG. 211.—Female pelvis (adult).

fig. 26

There are variances between male and female pelvises that can make a big difference in our yoga practice. The female pelvis is sometimes referred to as the obstetrics pelvis. Evolutionary changes in the pelvis allowed woman to carry and deliver children safely while still being able to ambulate. For this reason, the female pelvis will have a larger, flared ilia and pelvic inlet. The pubic arch for a woman is generally greater than 90 degrees, while a male pubic arch is generally less than 90 degrees. A female acetabulum presents more anteriorly medial while a male acetabulum presents more laterally. This allows men to walk by bringing their legs forward, with minimal swing of the pelvis and abduction of the femurs. Because of the direction of their hip sockets, women have a greater swing to their pelvis, and have to abduct their femurs more. By reviewing what you have learned from the last chapter about the differences in the male and female sacrum and sacroiliac joint, you can see that a woman's pelvis has more movement and flexibility but will suffer more instability and potential injury to the SI joints, where as men's pelvises are more stable and congruent, but will have less mobility and flexibility. Also, because of the presentation of the hip sockets, even disregarding the flexibility of the surrounding muscles, women will often be able to come into a cross-legged seat and have their knees closer to the floor than men.

♀ Built for
♂ babies

Think of your pelvis as a bowl full of soy chai latte. This is what I'm currently drinking right now, but please feel free to imagine your own favorite beverage. If you tip the bowl forward, all of your chai will fall out anteriorly. This is called an anterior tilt. The ASIS will move inferiorly, and your ischial tuberosities will move posteriorly as if you are trying to show off your booty. If you tip the bowl backwards, all your yummy chai will spill out posteriorly. This is called a posterior tilt. The ASIS will move superiorly, and your tail and ischial tuberosities will tuck under. This will make you look like a scared dog, or like you are trying out your best pelvic thrust dance moves. Because of some prevalent muscular imbalances and habits, I think we usually fall into 1 of these 2 camps: a booty popper, or a pelvic thruster. Both misalignments are not efficient and put the back, hips, and knees in jeopardy. Pulling the flesh out from behind your sitting bones, or sitting on your tailbone like the kickstand of a bicycle both tend to misalign the pelvis in our seated postures, and then everything on top and below the pelvis goes wonky. Finding balance in the bowl of the pelvis often means the coccyx and pubic bone will be equidistant to the floor.

then should we

Let's do a taste test:

I've heard this before

Come to stand in tadasana, or mountain pose. Place your feet hip-distance apart with your feet facing forward. Soften your knees so they don't have to be locked, and roll your inner thigh flesh back. Deepen and soften your hip crease (inguinal crease) and relax your tush muscles. Do a little hula dance between the two extremes of booty popping and pelvic thrusting. Come to the place of balance where you feel the pubic bone and tailbone parallel to the floor. Apply light engagement of the lower abdomen as you lengthen the spine upwards, making sure to keep the hip crease and tush muscles relaxed.

Femur

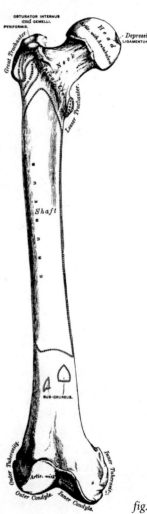

fig. 27

Yay femur! It's got it all!

The femur wins the prize for being the longest bone in the body. Its femoral head articulates with the acetabulum (hip socket) making a classic ball and socket joint. A ball and socket joint enjoys the most freedom of movement. The femur can move in all three planes at the hip socket, taking flexion, extension, abduction, adduction, external and internal rotation and circumduction (circular movement). It is deeply congruent, and often said to be analogous with an orange sitting inside a coffee cup. The deep snugly fit of the joint, the large muscles, sheets of ligaments, and connective tissue that surround the joint make this a very strong and stable area.

The femoral head tapers slightly at the neck of the femur before meeting the two prominences called the greater trochanter and lesser trochanter. Any lumps or bumps on a bone are a great place for muscle attachment. The greater trochanter can be felt on the lateral side of the hip if you place your hand on the outer thigh and rotate your femur bone. The lesser trochanter is deep under many thick muscles and is very hard to palpate. Moving distally, we have the long shaft of the femur which converges medially towards the knee. This angle can vary ("knock kneed" or "bow legged") but is generally greater in women because of our wider-set pelvis. On the distal end of the femur, we have two oblong eminences known as the condyles (medial and lateral). In between these lower lumps, we have a smooth shallow articular depression called the patellar surface, the groove in which the patella slides.

Patella

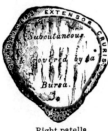
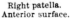
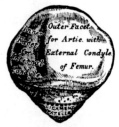

Right patella.
Anterior surface.

Right patella.
Posterior surface.

fig. 28

The patella, or kneecap, is a sesamoid bone, or a bone that forms inside of a tendon sheath. The patella develops inside the quadriceps tendon around the age of 2. I often palpate my friends' small children's knees to see and celebrate the ossification of this small bone. The patella provides some protection to the knee joint, but its primary role is to amplify the leverage that the tendon can exert on the femur, giving you more bang for the buck in knee extension.

Tibia

The tibia, or shinbone, is the larger of the two lower leg bones. It articulates with the femur, making what's called the "true knee joint" (the patella and fibula are considered accessory bones). Its somewhat sharp edge can be felt on the anterior surface of the shin. The large bump that you can palpate below your patella on your tibia is called the tibial tuberosity. The distal end of the tibia is seen and felt as the inner bump (medial malleolus) on your ankle.

Fibula

Like a fib is a small lie, the fibula is the smaller, more delicate of your lower leg

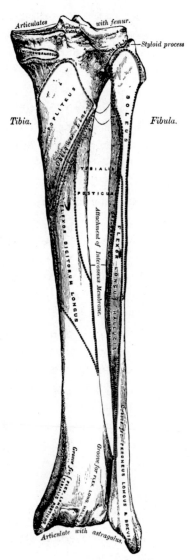

fig. 28

bones. Found on the lateral aspect of your lower leg, it forms a superior and inferior joint with the tibia and a distal articulation with your talus (ankle joint). This bone is difficult to feel on the lateral aspect of your shin, but can best be seen and felt as the outer bump (lateral malleolus) on your ankle.

The ankle joint

The medial and lateral malleolus grasp the talus like a monkey wrench, making the snug hinge joint of the ankle. The actions of the ankle joint are named slightly different than the movements that come from the bones and joints above. When we point our foot like a dancer, we are plantar flexing our ankle. When we draw the toes back toward the front of our shin, we are dorsiflexing our ankle. The other movements that we observe in our ankle like inversion (rolling to the outside of the foot) or eversion (rolling to the inside edge of the foot) are a combination of movements from the other tarsal and metatarsal bones.

The foot and arches

Containing 26 bones, 33 joints, and more than 100 muscles, tendons, and ligaments, the foot is a stunning piece of architecture. The large calcaneus, or heel bone, is designed to bear the brunt of the weight and heel strike during walking. The other large, rock-like tarsals take up nearly half the foot and help to distribute the weight and force while standing and walking. The teeny tiny phalanges (toes) act to fine tune balance and help to propel us forward during the push off phase of walking.

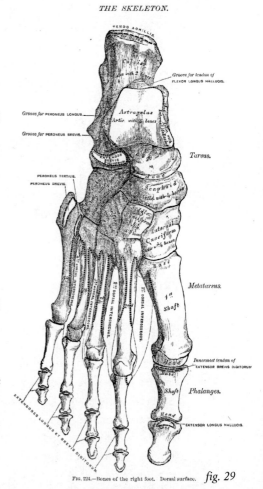

THE SKELETON.

Fig. 234.—Bones of the right foot. Dorsal surface. *fig. 29*

If you look at the plantar side of your foot (sole) you can see it has three distinguishable arches: a medial, lateral and transverse arch. The most impressive of these arches is the medial arch, the second place winner is the transverse arch, and bringing up the rear, the lateral arch. These arches act as shock absorbers and help magnify the force generated when we walk. As we walk, we are meant to heel strike, then transfer weight to the pinky side of the foot (up the lateral arch). Then, our foot rolls toward the distal end of our first metatarsal (below the big toe), moving across the transverse arch. We then are able to push off from the big toe using the large medial arch to generate more amplified force without a ton of muscular energy.

Supporting these arches is a thick layer of plantar fascia that runs from the calcaneus to the heads of the metatarsals. This is a frequent site of injury and irritation which can manifest as plantar fasciitis. Often, our feet, trapped in shoes, forget they have these arches and muscular support, which may contribute to this tissue getting irritated. Hopefully, by using these arches in our yoga practice, we strengthen the muscles in the foot and help to reintegrate the intelligence and mobility of this structure.

Preventing plantar fasciitis

SOME OF THE MUSCLES IN THE NEIGHBORHOOD

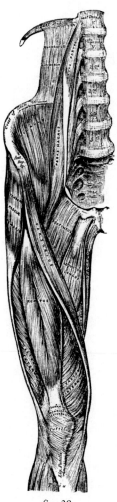

You can imagine your hip and leg as if they are divided into 4 quadrants: a front compartment, back compartment, inner compartment, and outer compartment. For the most part, when the front compartment contracts, the hip flexes. When the back compartment contracts, the hip extends. The inner compartment contracts, causing adduction, and the outer compartment contracts, causing abduction.

If you think about the last 7 days of your life (quickly please), chances are you might notice much more flexion in the hip (sitting at your desk or in the car), external rotation (the legs tend to fall and walk slightly externally rotated), and abduction (from both walking and sitting). This imbalance in action will often bring an imbalance to the muscles, and can compromise the neutrality of the pelvis and function of the knees. If you think of the last 7 yoga classes you have taken, unfortunately, chances are these same imbalances were emphasized, as we tend to work more with forward bends (flexion at the hip), turning our legs out, and abducting. If we can become more conscious of this and purposefully add in more extension, adduction, and internal rotation at the hip, we can help to bring about a sweeter balance.

Thoughtful yoga practice can counteract the common movements that create imbalance in our everyday life

fig. 30

Hip Flexors

Psoas

The psoas is the prime mover of flexion at the hip joint. This muscle has attachments to the transverse processes and bodies of vertebrae T12-L5. It runs anterior to the pelvis and attaches to the lesser trochanter of the femur. The psoas joins up with a muscle called the iliacus, which is on the anterior surface of the ilia and shares a tendon and attachment to the femur. For this reason, the muscles are sometimes talked about together and referred to as the iliopsoas.

The psoas contracts when the femur is in flexion at the hip, like the when we bring our knees into our chest. We help to stretch the psoas when we extend the femur at the hip, like the back leg in our lunge pose.

Quadriceps Femoris

The quadriceps are actually 4 muscles with a common insertion on the tibial tuberosity.

Vastus lateralis, vastus medialis, and vastus intermedius originate on the femur and cross the knee joint, acting only as extensors of the knee

Rectus femoris originates on the anterior inferior iliac spine (smaller bump on ilia, inferior to the ASIS), crosses both the hip joint and the knee joint, and acts as a hip flexor and a knee extensor.

All 4 of these muscles come together at the patellar tendon. This tendon encapsulates the patella and attaches to the tibial tuberosity. This is why as you sit on the floor with your legs stretched out in front of you and contract and release your quadriceps, you can watch the patella slide up and down the patellar groove. You should also be able to grasp your patella and carefully wiggle it slightly side to side when the quadriceps are relaxed.

The 3 vastus sisters and rectus femoris are contracted when we extend our knee and the rectus femoris is contracted when we flex the femurs at the hip joint. When we take our "standing, hold the big toe posture" or hasta padagustasana, we are contracting the lifted legs quadriceps group. To stretch these muscles, we can take extension at the hip (rectus femoris) and flexion of the knee (3 vastus sisters) like the back leg in our dreaded "King Arthur pose" where we lunge with the back knee down, then attempt to lift the back heel towards our tush. Oy vey!

get on the floor and find these when you forget

Sartorius

The sartorius is the longest muscle in the body. Its name translates as "tailor's muscle" referring to the way tailors used to sit cross-legged on the floor to hem pants. This muscle takes on a snake-like appearance as it originates on the ASIS and sweeps across the thigh, attaching to the upper medial tibia. Since this muscle crosses both the hip joint and the knee, it will have action on both joints. When contracted, it will flex and abduct the hip, externally rotate the thigh, and flex the knee joint. Just like our tailor friends, yogis utilize this muscle when trying to sit in a cross-legged position as well as in many poses that use this very familiar action. We are helping to stretch this muscle when we extend, internally rotate, or adduct the femur at the hip joint and extend the knee.

Hip Extensors

Hamstrings

The hamstrings are 3 muscles that act together to extend the hip joint and flex the knee joint.

Semimembranosus and semitendinosus originate on the ischial tuberosities and attach to the medial side of the tibia.

Biceps femoris originates on the ischial tuberosities and attaches to the lateral aspect of the fibula.

You can feel these tendons at the back of your knee. They often feel like banjo strings on either side of your knee crease.

We contract the hamstrings to bring the legs into extension at the hip and flexion in our knees, like in bow pose (dhanurasana).

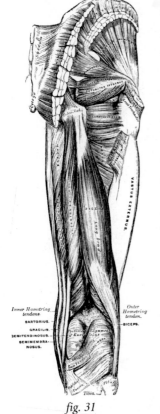

fig. 31

We stretch the hamstrings when we find flexion at the hip and extension at the knee, like in our standing forward bend pose (uttanasana).

Gluteus Maximus

The gluteus maximus muscle is the largest muscle in the body. It is the prime mover in extension at the hip. It originates on the posterior side of the ilium and sacrum and attaches to the gluteal tuberosity on the superior-lateral aspect of the femur and the iliotibial band (IT band). While extension of the hip is its primary job, as a side job it will also perform external rotation of the femur. We contract this muscle when we bring our leg into extension or external rotation, like a dancer might in the back leg of her arabesque. We help to stretch this muscle when we flex or internally rotate the femur, like in our forward bending poses with "pigeon toes".

who knew?

Often in our back bending postures (like bridge, wheel, or bow pose), we are bringing the femurs into extension at the hip joint. Because the gluteus maximus is the prime mover of that action, it fires up and does its side job of external rotation, too. This is why you might notice a tendency to roll your thighs and knees open in these postures. While this may bring you deeper or higher into the pose, it also will grip the sacroiliac joints and jam the lumbar spine. This is why teachers often tell you to relax your tush. While the gluteus maximus will still be firing, we can turn the muscular volume down and fine-tune the action with the hamstrings and the adductors. Placing a block between your thighs will help you get to know these muscles and create more space in lower spine.

Hip Abductors

The hip abductors stabilize the pelvis and help to keep it aligned when we support weight on one foot. They contract with every step you take, and therefore tend to be much stronger and hyper-contracted than the adductor group.

Gluteus Medius and Minimus

These two fan-shaped muscles are deep to the gluteus maximus. They originate on the outer cavity of the posterior ilium and insert on the greater trochanter of the femur. They both help to abduct the femur and to stabilize the pelvis when walking. When the femur is flexed at the hip, they also act as internal rotators, helping to balance the strong external rotation component of the gluteus maximus.

Tensor Fascia Lata

This is one of my favorite muscles because it sounds like a drink you would order at

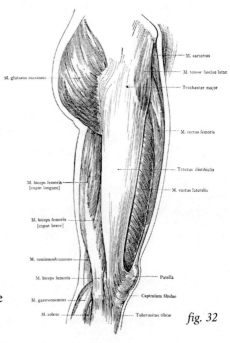

fig. 32

Starbucks. It originates on the iliac crest near the ASIS and inserts on the iliotibial band. The IT band is a strong rope of connective tissue that runs down the lateral aspect of the thigh and inserts on the lateral tibia and head of the fibula, helping to stabilize the outer leg. The tensor fascia lata abducts and internally rotates the femur.

Hip Adductors

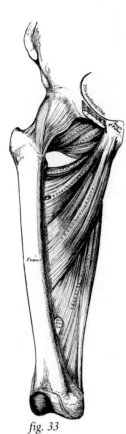

fig. 33

The hip adductors help to draw the thighs together to the midline or across the midline. Because of some of our habitual tendencies, they are often underutilized and weak. We can draw awareness to these muscles by trying to isometrically draw our legs together in our standing poses. We also can fire them strongly when trying to do our arm balancing and inverting postures to help us become more stable.

Pectineus, Adductor Brevis, and Adductor Longus

These muscles originate on the pubis and insert on the linea aspera, a ridge on the posterior aspect of the femur. They adduct the femur

Adductor Magnus

This large (hence, "magnus") muscle originates on the ischial tuberosities and the pubis and attaches to the linea aspera. Because of its more posterior nature, it also acts as an extensor and an adductor of the femur at the hip.

Gracilis

The gracilis originates on the pubis and inserts on the medial tibia. Because this muscle crosses both the hip and knee joint, it will have action on both joints. In addition to adduction of the femur, it also flexes the knee.

External Rotators of the Hip

There are 6 deep external rotators of the hip joint in addition to the strong external rotation of the gluteus maximus.

6 External Rotators

Gemellus Superior, Gemellus Inferior, Obturator Internus, Obturator Externus and Quadratus Femoris

These muscles all originate on the pelvis, deep to the gluteals, and insert on the greater trochanter of the femur. In addition to external rotation of the femur, they provide a sort of hammock for supporting the pelvis. When the femur is fixed, like in our standing poses, these muscles can help to lift the pelvis slightly away from the femur, allowing for more space in the hip joint.

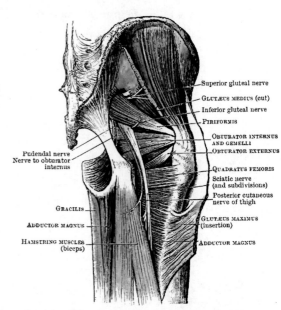

fig. 34 THE MUSCLES AND NERVES OF THE RIGHT BUTTOCK.

5 Piriformis

The piriformis originates on the anterior surface of the sacrum and attaches to the greater trochanter. This external rotator often gets a bum rap. The large sciatic nerve (about the size of a highlighter pen) runs just posterior to this muscle, and for a small minority of people, runs through this muscle. Because we tend to externally rotate quite a bit, this muscle can become hyper-contracted and press on the sciatic nerve, causing sharp, shooting nerve pain, or sciatica. The sciatic branch is a large nerve derived from spinal nerves L4-S3. This means that it has many opportunities to get annoyed, and is not always piriformis' fault. Disc problems in the lower lumbar spine, sacroiliac dysfunction, and a myriad of muscle tightness all can apply pressure to the sciatic branch, causing sciatica.

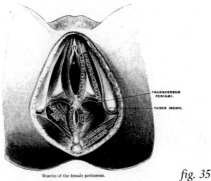

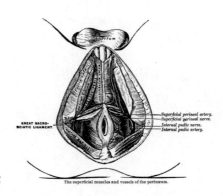

fig. 35

6 Pelvic Floor

The pelvic floor, or pelvic diaphragm, is a sling of overlapping muscles that help to support the weight of the pelvic organs, assist in urinary and fecal continence, aid in sexy time, stabilize connecting joints, and act as a venous and lymphatic pump for the pelvis. We can experience movement of this pelvic diaphragm with our breath. As we inhale, our bodies will literally conspire to accommodate this inspiration. The pelvic floor softens and draws slightly inferior. On exhalation, this diaphragm rises superior and can even be contracted upward to help give us a little extra oomph and support. Like any other muscle group, we would like these muscles to be both strong and supple.

Males have 2 openings and females have 3 openings to the external environment in this pelvic diaphragm. This means that the female pelvic floor will, by nature, have more flexibility, but will usually be weaker than a male pelvic floor. Conversely, a male pelvic floor will usually be a little less flexible. Carrying extra weight, pregnancy, childbirth, and gravity's pull on our organs over time will all contribute to a weakening to this region. We can help strengthen these muscles by including them in our deep exhales and the practice of mula bandha (root lock).

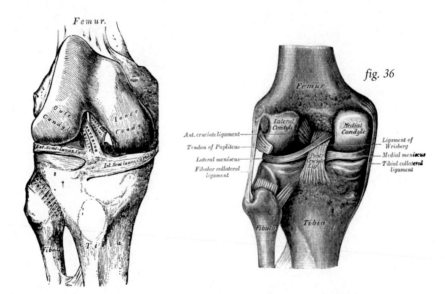

fig. 36

The Knee Joint

The "true" knee joint is the articulation of the femur and the tibia. This joint is considered a gliding hinge joint and will perform flexion and extension.

The femur glides a little bit like a rocking horse forward on the tibia during flexion and backwards on extension. The femur will also slightly spiral externally upon flexion and internally spiral upon extension of the knee. While there is slight spiraling available in this joint, it does not rotate. It's important that we do not ask or force rotation in this joint because it can cause some serious damage to the joint and surrounding tissues.

To support the alignment of these two bones in relation to one another, we have four ligaments. The medial and lateral collateral ligaments keep the knee from displacing from side to side. The anterior and posterior cruciate ligaments help keep the knee from displacing forward and backward. Inside the joint we have two special discs of fibrocartilage called the meniscus. They help to deepen the congruency of the joint as well as provide cushioning and absorb shock.

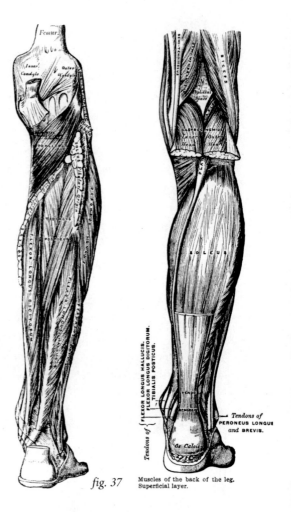

fig. 37

Muscles of the back of the leg. Superficial layer.

Keeping the knee healthy must pay attention to how we are rotating it!

SOME OF THE MUSCLES IN THE NEIGHBORHOOD

Popliteus

The popliteus is a small muscle on the posterior side of the knee joint. It "unlocks" the knee in flexion and helps to stabilize and protect the knee joint in our squatting postures.

Gastrocnemius

The gastrocnemius, or calf muscle, originates on the posterior bumps (or condyles) on the lower aspect of the femur and inserts on the calcaneus by way of the Achilles' tendon. Because it crosses both the knee and ankle, it will have action on both joints. It brings about flexion of the knee and plantar flexion of the ankle.

Peroneals

Found in the lateral compartment of the lower leg this muscle acts to evert the foot and plantar flex the ankle.

Tibialis Anterior

Situated on the lateral side of the tibia, this muscle inverts the foot and dorsiflexes the ankle.

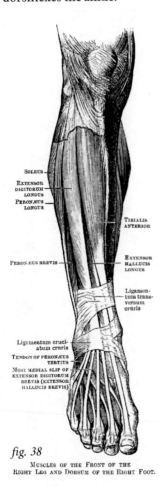

fig. 38

MUSCLES OF THE FRONT OF THE
RIGHT LEG AND DORSUM OF THE RIGHT FOOT.

Chapter 7

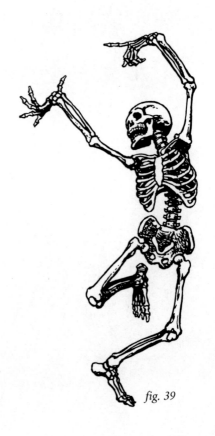

fig. 39

All Up In Arms
ANATOMY OF THE UPPER LIMB

"Dance is bigger than the physical body. When you extend your arm, it doesn't stop at the end of your fingers, because you're bigger than that; you're dancing spirit"

- JUDITH JAMISON

How we carry our shoulders in life speaks volumes to those around us. Are we carrying the weight of the world on our shoulders? Are our shoulders anxiously hunched up by our ears? Think of the classic depressed posture with the shoulders slumped, or a bad actor overdramatizing on stage with the shoulders drawn far back and the chest protruding forward. Even if we don't know the anatomy, we know how to read this energy.

The alignment of these highly mobile joints becomes even more important to us when we decide to place weight on them in our yoga practice. We have evolved to bear weight and walk on our lower limbs. Our upper limbs allow us to climb, carry, hold, and manipulate objects with great precision (I don't mean texting). This means that our arms and hands, structurally speaking, are poorly equipped to support our weight. If we do decide to support our weight with our upper limbs, we must employ other intelligence and muscles in the area to help make this safer and more efficient.

Scapula

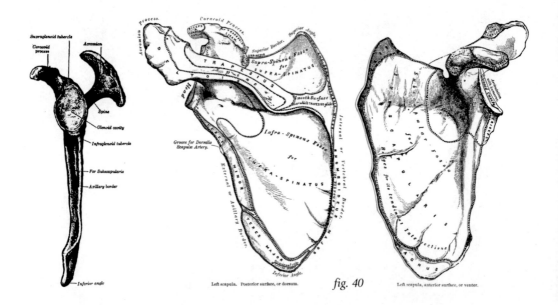

fig. 40

The scapulae, or shoulder blades, are two triangular-shaped bones found on the posterior side of the ribcage. Looking at the posterior aspect of the scapula, we observe the superior border (top), medial border (closer to the spine), and axillary border (fancy word for armpit side). The three angles of the triangle are called the superior, inferior, and lateral.

On the lateral aspect of the scapula is the glenoid fossa, or socket, which will

form an articulation with the head of the humerus, making the highly
mobile ball and socket joint. Just like the other ball and socket joint, the hip,
it has flexion, extension, abduction, adduction, external and internal
rotation, and circumduction on its resumé. While the hip joint is sometimes
said to be analogous to an orange sitting inside a coffee cup, the glenohumeral
joint (shoulder joint) is more like an orange sitting on a coffee cup saucer.
This means that there is less surface area of the humerus touching the
glenoid fossa, and much less congruency. Again, because we, in life, are not
meant to support our weight on our arms, we have evolved a highly moveable and thusly less stable shoulder joint.

It is important to mention that when the scapula are in anatomical position,
the sockets do not face straight out to the sides, but rather slightly forward
at an angle. In yoga, we often emphasize "drawing your shoulders back" so
much that we unwittingly create a new "neutral" that has our shoulders by
our sides, or even back behind us. This is just as unnatural, and possibly as
injurious as slumping the shoulders forward.

The costal, or rib, side of the scapula is smooth and curved, and glides over
the ribcage with no bony attachment or joint. This allows the scapula
to have the additional movements of elevation (shrugging your shoulders
towards your ears), depression (drawing the scapulae down your back),
protraction (scapulae move laterally away from one another), retraction
(scapulae move medially towards one another), upward rotation (inferior
angle will rotate upwards), downward rotation (inferior angle will rotate
downwards), anterior tipping (tips anteriorly), and posterior tipping (tips
posteriorly). This adds even more mobility to the already quite mobile
shoulder joint.

A process that can be seen projecting anteriorly from the scapula is the
coracoid process. Coracoid means "crow's beak" and can often be felt on
the anterior chest near the shoulder. Like all pointy pieces of a bone, it will
serve as a great place for muscle attachment.

On the posterior side of the shoulder blade is a bony ridge called the spine
of the scapula. It rises up and forms an awning on top of the shoulder called
the acromion process. The acromion will articulate with the clavicle at
the acromioclavicular, or AC joint. Like every other bone in the body, the
scapulae and the acromion processes are wildly different for each of us.
The size of the acromion and how much it overhangs the shoulder joint
makes a real difference to the amount of movement available in your
shoulders. In this case, size really does matter. If you have an acromion that

overhangs the joint, you may not be able to bring your arms up to frame your ears like your teacher is asking of you, or you might not be able to bring them behind the ears to attempt wheel pose. This has to be ok. Another reason why as teachers we cannot assume the same exact shape for each lovely unique student.

At this point, I usually make my students take a pledge. Please repeat after me:

"I, (state your name), do solemnly swear to always ask for external rotation of my humerus before I ask it to do flexion! So help me Shiva!"

While this may seem silly, when we externally rotate our humerus, we have a better shot at bypassing the acromion process in the act of humeral flexion, and may even head off any rubbing or grinding (get your mind out of the gutter) of the tissues that are in the neighborhood.

Clavicle

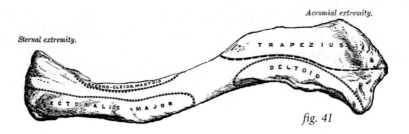

fig. 41

These 2 S-shaped bones form the only bony attachment of the upper limb to the axial skeleton. The medial end articulates with the top part of the sternum at the sternoclavicular joint. The lateral end articulates with the scapula at the acromioclavicular joint. You can feel, and often see, this V-shaped joint on the top of your shoulder where you might throw the strap of your bag. A separated shoulder will often refer to a separation or dislocation of the AC joint.

Humerus

The humerus, or upper arm bone, is the long bone that runs from the shoulder to the elbow. Proximally, its head articulates with the glenoid fossa of the scapula (glenohumeral joint). Like the other synovial joints that we have mentioned, it has all the bells and whistles like ligaments, joint capsules, synovial fluid, and a special piece of fibrocartilage called a labrum. Just like the labrum in the hip joint, this ring of cartilage - like a washer you would see inside your faucet - helps to create a more congruent fit. Distally,

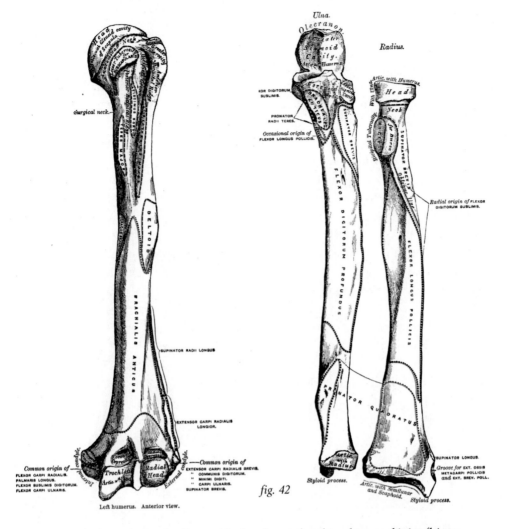

fig. 42

Left humerus. Anterior view.

the humerus articulates with the ulna at the ulnar-humeral joint (hinge joint of the elbow) and the radius with a gliding joint called the radio-humeral joint.

Ulna

In anatomical position, the ulna is the medial pinky-side forearm bone. It articulates with the humerus at the elbow joint. It has a hook-like projection that you can feel on the posterior side of the elbow that sits in the notch at the distal end of the humerus. You might have had the experience of "hitting your funny bone." When the elbow is flexed, this notch is exposed as well as a nerve that runs along side of it called the ulnar nerve. Because this nerve is very near to the surface, it is occasionally hit, producing that not-so-funny sensation.

The ulna also articulates proximally and distally with the radius, and distally with the carpals at the wrist.

Radius

In anatomical position, the lateral or thumb-side forearm bone is called the radius. The radius, like its name suggests, can radiate, or roll over the ulna. These movements are named supination (palm would face up like you're holding a cup of soup) and pronation (like you would "pro it" - or throw it - to the floor). We all have a different amount of pronation available to us. As a test, create a 90-degree angle at your elbow joint (flexion). Holding the upper arm still, pronate your palm. If the palm is not parallel to the floor, the humerus will have to internally rotate to make that happen. We ask for pronation of the palms in downward facing dog. If you are limited in forearm pronation, you will be forced to internally rotate your humerus while you are in flexion at the shoulder. You took a very legally binding oath earlier to assure me you would not do this! Modifications must be made to the pose to prevent injury to the shoulder. Coming down on your forearms and interlacing your fingers in downward facing dog or changing up the pose entirely might be ways to lessen stress on the shoulder joint.

The radius articulates with the humerus, participating in the hinge joint of the elbow, as well as a proximal and distal articulation with the ulna. Its distal end will also articulate with the carpals at the wrist joint.

Wrist and Hands

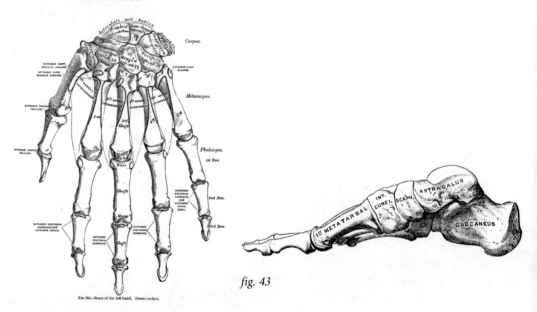

fig. 43

The bones of the hands are very similar to the bones of the feet. In the feet, we have the rock-like tarsus, the long metatarsals, and the phalanges. In the hands, we have the pebble-like carpals, long metacarpals, and the phalanges.

If you look, though, you will notice the tarsus of the feet make up nearly one-half of the foot length, and the puny, but oh-so-cute, phalanges make up merely one-fourth. Conversely, in the hands, the teeny tiny carpals barely take up one-fourth of the hand length, but the long phalanges make up nearly one-half. This is because we are meant to bear weight on the large tarsus of the feet, and we push off and refine balance using our toes. Bearing weight on our hands can be done, of course, but keep in mind their structure is not well suited for it.

On the palmar side of the wrist, you have a strong sheet of connective tissue called the flexor retinaculum. Like Saran Wrap over a bowl of spaghetti, it helps to hold the tendons and nerves that run through the tunnel made by the curved placement of the two rows of carpals. Our modern lives tend to bring in a lot of congestion into our hands and wrists. Using the keyboard and mouse on your computer, as well as texting and holding our phones, brings a claw-like hand into our yoga practice. Repeated claw-like action during our day causes the nerves that pass deep to this tissue to compress, leading to pain, numbness, or tingling of the fingers (carpal tunnel syndrome). Yoga can definitely be a tonic to help stretch and open these tissues, but it also can be the cause of injury to the wrist due to all of this weight bearing on our hands. When beginning a yoga practice, it is best to minimize the amount of time trying to support weight on your hands. As you begin to gain more awareness and openness in the arms and shoulders, you can build up your time spent here. Also, before you place weight on your hands, line up your wrist creases (wrinkles made in the front of the wrist by extension) parallel to the front edge of your mat. Because of our unique anatomy, this may mean that your fingers are forward, or maybe radiated slightly open. Spreading out through your long fingers to pour the weight evenly through your hands while you draw up through the forearm muscles will also help to distribute the weight from the wrists.

The Rotator Cuff Muscles

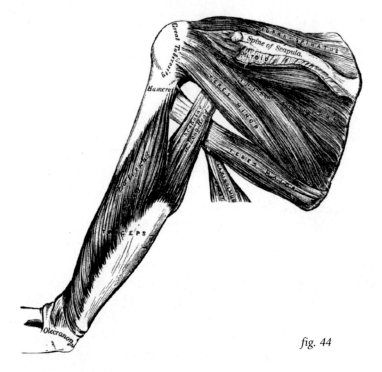

fig. 44

The rotator cuff muscles are a group of 4 muscles which all have their bodies on the scapula and attach to the head of the humerus. Their main job is to keep the wildly mobile head of the humerus in the socket of the scapula. They surround the joint on three sides and have their own distinct actions.

Supraspinatus

Supraspinatus is found on the posterior side of the scapula, above the spine of the scapula. This muscle dives inferior to the acromion process before attaching to the head of the humerus and will initiate arm abduction. Out of all 4 rotator cuff muscles, this one is the most frequently injured. Supraspinatus tendonitis, tearing, or sub-acromial bursitis (irritation to the bursa underneath the acromion) are common problems that can rise up in a yoga practice when we don't follow our oath about externally rotating our arms before flexion. It's easy to run the humerus into the acromion process and wear or irritate these tissues. When this muscle is "off-line" the deltoid (shoulder cap) muscle will often take over in the act of arm abduction and give your student a shrugged-shoulder appearance.

Infraspinatus

Infraspinatus is found on the posterior side of the scapula below the spine of the scapula. It will help to externally rotate the humerus.

Teres Minor

This muscle originates on the lateral border of the scapula and assists in external rotation of the humerus.

Subscapularis

This is found on the anterior surface of the scapula and attaches to the head of the humerus. When contracted, it will internally rotate and adduct the humerus.

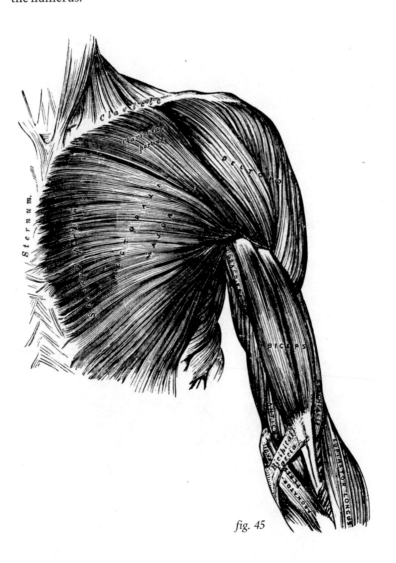

fig. 45

Pectoralis Major

This muscle originates on the sternum and the costal cartilage of ribs 2-6 and attaches to the upper humerus. The tendon can be felt in the anterior axilla (armpit). I sometimes refer to it as the hugging muscle because it flexes, adducts, and internally rotates your humerus like you would do if you were to reach out and hug someone.

Latissimus Dorsi

The latissimus dorsi muscle is a large posterior muscle that originates from the lower thoracic, lumbar, sacral vertebra, illiac crest, and thoraco-lumbar fascia and attaches to the upper humerus. When contracted, it will adduct, extend, and internally rotate the humerus. We use this muscle when drawing the chest forward or open in our upward facing dog pose.

Deltoid

This is what you would think of as the muscular cap or shoulder pad on top of your shoulder. Its teardrop shape has anterior, medial, and posterior fibers that originate on the clavicle, acromion, and spine of the scapula and attach to the deltoid tuberosity of the humerus. This small lump can be felt on the lateral aspect of the humerus. When this muscle contracts, it can flex, abduct, and extend the humerus.

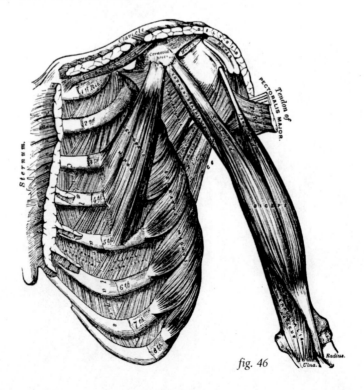

fig. 46

Serratus Anterior

Just like the serrated knife in your kitchen, this muscle has small finger-like projections that originate on the superior border of the first 9 ribs and slide underneath the scapula to attach to its medial border. When contracted, it helps to upwardly rotate and protract your scapula. If you have ever witnessed someone doing a yoga push up (chaturanga dandasana) and noticed the medial border of their scapula "winging" or lifting off their ribs, chances are the serratus anterior muscle is weak or not engaged.

Pectoralis Minor

Pectoralis minor is deep to petoralis major and originates on the superior margins of ribs 3-5 and inserts on the coracoid process of the scapula. When contracted, it can anteriorly tip the scapula or assist in breathing by lifting these ribs for a greater inspiration.

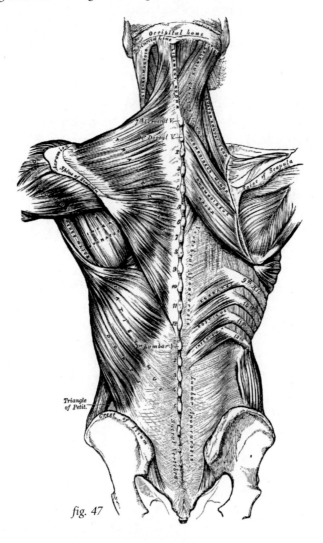

fig. 47

Levator Scapula

Originating on the transverse processes of C1-C4, it attaches to the superior angle of the scapula and elevates the scapula, as well as laterally flexes and rotates the cervical spine.

Rhomboids

Almost looking like a Christmas tree, these muscles originate from the spinous processes of C7-T5 and attach to the medial border of the scapula. Their big job is retraction of the scapula.

Trapezius

The trapezius is a large diamond-shaped superficial muscle on the posterior side of the body. It originates from the occiput (base of the skull) and cervical/thoracic spinous processes and attaches to the clavicle, acromion, and spine of the scapula. Because it is such a vast muscle, different fibers will elevate, depress, upwardly rotate, downwardly rotate, and retract the scapula.

The typical poor postural habit that I see in my students is a sunken chest and the shoulders hunched forward up by the ears. We know this affects our mood, energy, and breath, but it will also have very real and negative repercussions for our shoulders when coming into our postures. In this postural pitfall, the pectoralis major and minor will be very contracted, pulling the humerus forward and into internal rotation (remember your oath?). This contraction will also anteriorly tip the scapula. The rhomboids and serratus anterior will be underutilized and weak, providing even less "muscular glue" for the scapula on the back. Think of trying to push something heavy away from you. You will be stronger if you keep the scapula on the back rather than if you let them drift off the sides of the ribs. When doing the heavy lifting of our own body weight in the yoga practice, this poor posture will unfortunately contribute to injury in and around the shoulder joint. We are best served by opening the front of the chest and strengthening the muscles that support the scapula on the back before we try to move through the heavy lifting of our postures.

Chapter 8

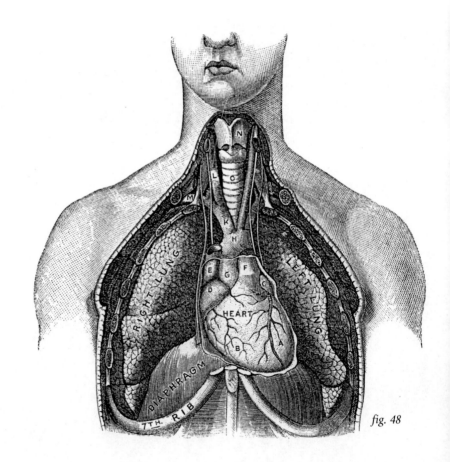

fig. 48

It's Right Under Your Nose
THE BEAUTY AND POTENTIAL OF YOUR BREATH

"I take refuge in the breath.
Breath is all this, whatever there
is, and all that ever will be.
I take refuge in the breath."

- CHANDOGYA UPANISHAD

Atman is the arrow
Prana is the bow
Brahman the target

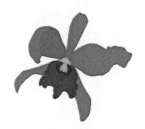

- UPANISHADS

It might be easy to overlook or underestimate the power of the breath. Right now, giving it no thought at all, throwing it no well-deserved party, the breath is delivering 11,000 liters of air to you every day. That's enough to fill 10 million balloons in a lifetime! This breath takes a circuitous path through 1,500 miles of airways in your lungs and 62,000 miles of circulatory system. All of this led by the commander - the heart - which selflessly beats, on average, 3 billion times in an average lifetime. Some of the old yogi texts state that we are given only a finite number of breaths in a lifetime, so it's best to slow them down and encourage each one to stick around in this body a little longer. Whether you believe this or not, harnessing the power of the breath can truly be transformative in your practice and your life.

The breath is controlled both by voluntary action as well as the autonomic nervous system. That means I could ask you right now to take a slower, deeper breath (go ahead, I'll wait) and you can oblige, but as you have been sitting here engrossed in this book, your body has taken care of the breath without your conscious help. Either way, the breath is initiated nervously (via the nervous system) by a muscle called the diaphragm. The diaphragm is sometimes likened to a portabella mushroom cap, an open umbrella, or my favorite, a jellyfish. The muscle circumnavigates and connects to the inside of the lower 6 ribs and has 2 tethers to the lumbar vertebrae. While as teachers and students of anatomy, we like to give clear origins and insertions for muscles and other tissues of the body; in reality, it's almost as arbitrary as the lines delineating the states in America. Some have obvious borders defined by mountains or rivers, but taking a larger view, everything is connected and interdependent. The diaphragm is a large muscle separating the thoracic (chest) and abdominal cavities and has interdidgetation (connection) to the psoas muscle and the tissues that hold and support the organs. The plura and pericardium (the connective tissue bags that hold the lungs and heart, respectively) are tied to the superior (top side) of the diaphragm. The peritoneal sac that envelops most of the abdominal organs is tied to the inferior (bottom side) of the diaphragm.

Whether the breath is initiated consciously or the body is taking care of the breath for you as you go about your business, the process remains the same. A nerve leading to your diaphragm fires and stimulates the diaphragm to contract. This causes the central tendon to pull downward, flattening towards the abdomen. This in turn creates a negative pressure in the thoracic cavity. Air loves to move to the area of lowest pressure, so air is funneled into the lungs via the nose or mouth, causing the lungs to expand. This might seem like a different view of respiration to you; it certainly did to me. I used to think that we very much sniffed the breath in and pushed

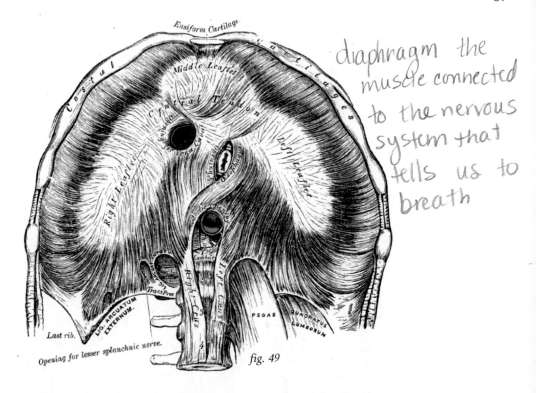

Ensiform Cartilage.

Middle Leaflet

Central Tendon

Right Leaflet

Left Leaflet

Oesophagus

Lumbar

Right Crus

Left Crus

Trans. Proc.

PSOAS

QUADRATUS LUMBORUM

LIG. ARCUATUM EXTERNUM.

Last rib.

Opening for lesser splanchnic nerve.

fig. 49

diaphragm the muscle connected to the nervous system that tells us to breath

the breath out. The real view is much more elegant, and dare I say, more
yogic. We really are just making space for the inspiration to pour into us as
if we are being breathed!

As the breath moves in and out, it takes a wondrous circuitous path through
the tubes and vessels of your form. Breathed in through the nostrils, air is
warmed and moistened as it travels past the mucosal membrane and small
cilia, or hair that lines the nose. It then ricochets through the cavernous
sinuses, creating a turbulence that further filters and warms the air. It takes
a 90-degree turn down the pharynx, then down the larynx, which contains
the vocal cords that can be narrowed or widened to draw the breath in
slower or faster. We purposely try to narrow the vocal folds to bring the
breath in slower in the pranayama technique ujjayi. I like to think of this
like drinking a really thick milkshake (frankly, because I love milkshakes)
through a longer, narrower straw. It will take a little more effort on your
part, but you can savor it for longer. From the larynx, the breath travels
down and branches into the two bronchi tubes on its way to the sponge-like
lungs. The breath then further branches off to 2, 4, 8...hundreds of thousands of smaller tributaries called bronchioles, which appear almost like 2
upside-down trees. At the end of these bronchioles rest what looks like a
dollhouse-sized miniature bunch of grapes, the alveoli. It's at the alveoli
which are flush with capillaries, that the exchange of oxygen and carbon
dioxide happens.

In the blood, the iron, or hemoglobin, proteins act almost like a horse (stay with me here). The oxygen molecule, much like a cowboy, jumps aboard and rides the hemoglobin through the arteries, into the smaller arterioles, and finally into the cell it desires to feed. The oxygen then jumps off, and the carbon dioxide hops aboard and travels back through the veins back to the heart and lungs for the recycling to begin. The carbon dioxide is then expelled through our exhalation. This tireless hemoglobin "horse" gallops through the system for nearly 120 days before moving to the spleen to retire.

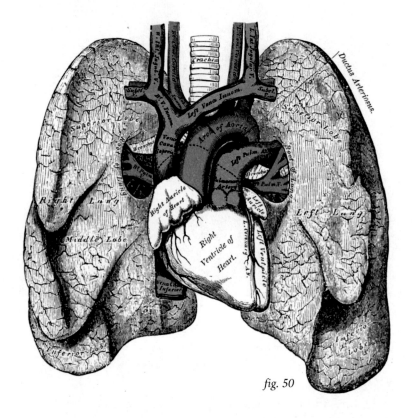

fig. 50

Although the diaphragm is what we call the prime mover of respiration, (the main muscle that does the job), other accessory muscles assist to help create more space for the breath. The abdominal muscles and pelvic floor soften and expand to give the organs, which are getting smushed by the diaphragm, a place to go. Some of your back muscles, like the erector spinae set and quadrates lumborum, contract to bring you into a small backbend and tug the lower ribs down. The muscles between your ribs, the internal and external intercostals, stretch and contract (respectively) to help open the bony cage around your lungs. You even have some neck muscles like the sternocleidomastoid and scalenes that helps to lift the collarbones and top few ribs to allow for the greatest expansion.

This may seem like a lot of fanfare for a simple breath but if you were to measure the surface area of all the nooks and crannies of your sponge-like lungs it would equal the size of a tennis court. This is some tremendous potential, and the body does what it can to help accommodate.

As you exhale, the diaphragm relaxes back into its domed shape towards the thoracic cavity. To help facilitate the exhalation, the abdominals and pelvic floor return back to their starting position, or contract. The erector spinae and quadratrus lumborum relax and lengthen, bringing you into a slightly rounded shape. The internal and external intercostals contract and expand (respectively) to soften the ribcage back in towards the center. The neck muscles relax, releasing the clavicles and sternum back to their neutral starting place. You can think of the muscular events that take place to help facilitate this breath as bringing us into the very smallest micro mini cow and cat pose. We take a very tiny backbend to help the inhalation and a very tiny rounding and softening in to help the exhalation. This is why in the yoga asana practice it feels more natural to follow the intelligence of the inhalation as we take postures that are lifting, expanding or back bending us, and exhaling as we find poses that fold, soften and return us back into our center.

One of my favorite quotes from the ancient yogic writings of The Kulanarva Tantra states, *"That which exists here - exists elsewhere, that which does not exist -exists nowhere."* It's one of those statements that you can ponder for a lifetime, but the way I begin to digest it is: the microcosm is a direct reflection of the macrocosm, and vice versa. So, I believe all of the esoteric pondering and yoga philosophy quoted by your favorite teachers have a physical resonance in the tissues of the body.

One thing that is often discussed in a yoga practice is the balance between engagement and surrender. In my experience, this is modeled beautifully by the biomechanics of our own anatomical breath. As we consciously and deeply breathe in our own yoga practice, through our engagement with the breath and the engagement or contraction of the diaphragm, our body literally conspires to make space for the inspiration to pour in. Depending on the shape or contortion we may be in, the breath moves to where there is space, and even begins to carve out space from the inside out. This begins to refine our concept of engagement being not one of control, per se, but rather engaging with the process without having dictate the experience.

With each inhale there is an opening, a stretch, a reach, a literal and ener-getic inspiration. There is a choice to engage with where you are and to follow the long loose tendrils of the breath as they unwind and slide into each nook and cranny. The exhale is a physical and energetic surrender. It is the yielding of the diaphragm, the belly, and the ribs towards your very center. It is a bowing to where you are and to what is. The surrender of whatever is tugging on your "mind's sleeve" to pull you away from the truth of where and who you are. The end of the exhale, at your most surrendered, is actually where you are the strongest, anatomically, and most primed for action. Physically, the belly and the pelvic floor can be at their most contracted. You are also at your lightest point. This is why in the vinyasa style of practice you often do all the "heavy lifting" of hopping or stepping forward at the end of the exhale. This also beautifully hints that the more you can surrender, soften, and become permeable, the stronger and more ready you are to receive the inrushing of inspiration that's just around the corner.

Chapter 9

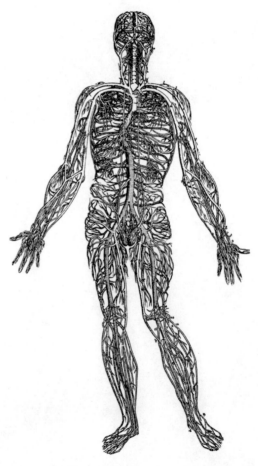

fig. 51

You've Got Some Nerve!

THE ELEGANT NERVOUS SYSTEM

"A single neuron may be rather dumb, but it is dumb in many subtle ways."

- FRANCIS CRICK

"How is it possible that a being with such sensitive jewels as the eyes, such enchanted musical instruments as the ears, and such fabulous arabesque of nerves as the brain can experience itself as anything less than a god."

- ALAN WATTS

Whoa! Wait! Look behind you! It's a tiger! Ok, so that was kind of mean, but you might notice now your pulse is racing, the body is shaking and sweating, and your breathing is labored. This is all due to the majestic nervous system! Even now as you are lifting and reading this book while breathing and digesting your lunch, you are under the nervous system's careful watch. The nervous system is our body's main control and communication center. Always striving to maintain homeostasis, it "talks" to every body system and activates muscles, glands, organs, and even thoughts to help bring you into a state of balance. Nerves are often referred to as the electrical wiring system of the body because they process and transfer information by means of nerve cells firing action potentials (electrical/chemical signals) which can zip along nerve fibers at speeds of up to 320 feet per second. There are 45 miles of nerves that map your body, but they can be arranged into a few different levels of organization.

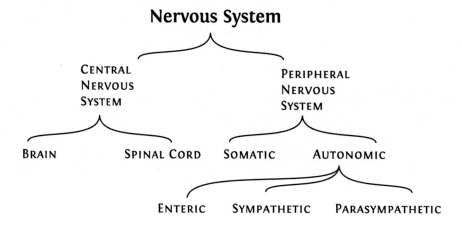

The Central Nervous System

The central nervous system (CNS) consists of the tissues of the brain and the spinal cord. Both of these wondrous tissues have the consistency of a firm tofu (ACK!), but luckily for us they have some layers of protection. The brain and spinal cord are protected most superficially by bone, three sheaths of tissue or meninges, and cerebral spinal fluid. The 3 or so pounds of brain matter sit in the bony vault of the skull, and the spinal cord, which runs continuous with this tissue, sits in the bony ring of the vertebral canal. The brain, our command center, can be divided into many different regions that we will explore more deeply in the next book (scenes from an upcoming attraction!). To wet your appetite though, I'll leave you with this mind blowing thought: the brain is made up of around 100 billion neurons. The number of synapses in the human brain is larger than the number of galaxies in the observable universe, even more than there are stars in our Milky Way galaxy. Each neuron has up to 100 thousand dendrites making over 100 trillion constantly changing connections. There are more potential ways to connect the brain's neurons than there are atoms in the universe (go ahead Google it, I'll wait...and look up Professor V.S. Ramachandran while you are there). Crazy awesome, right?

The spinal cord is a cylindrical structure that occupies the vertebral canal, a cavity extending the length of the vertebral column. It is usually 16-18 inches long, on average, and, in adults, does not extend the full length of the vertebral column. In adults, the conus medullaris (lower end of the spinal cord) is usually located at the level of L1 or L2 vertebrae. Below this, the vertebral canal is occupied largely by the elongated rootlets of the cauda equine, or horse's tail (lumbar and sacral spinal nerves), which travel down to the lower levels before they exit from the canal.

If it's the nervous system, and it's not the brain and spinal cord, it's in the peripheral nervous system.

Peripheral Nervous System

The peripheral nervous system (PNS) is the part of the nervous system consisting of the nerves and ganglia that exist outside of the brain and spinal cord. These nerves exit the spine through the little side holes made in between the vertebrae and from the base of the brain. Its main function, as its tributaries map your entire form, is to act as a 2-way communication relay between your muscles, organs, and glands to the central nervous system. The peripheral nervous system can be further subdivided into the somatic nervous system and the autonomic nervous system.

Somatic Nervous System

The somatic nervous system comes from the root word soma, meaning body, and is often referred to as the voluntary nervous system. These are the motor and sensory nerves that map our system and are under our voluntary or conscious control. These nerves innervate your skeletal muscles and are the part of the peripheral nervous system that we use to intentionally move, dance, or shake a tail feather.

Autonomic Nervous System

The autonomic nervous system is sometimes referred to as the involuntary nervous system, but I believe the better term is autonomic. Autonomic comes from the word autonomy, which translates as "a law unto itself." Instead of thinking about this as involuntary, or part of you that has gone rogue and completely out of your control, we can see this as having autonomy, but completely influenced by internal and external factors. These nerves will help to regulate your smooth and cardiac muscles, organs and glands. The autonomic nervous system can be further subdivided into 3 categories: the enteric, sympathetic, and parasympathetic nervous systems.

Enteric Nervous System

The enteric nervous system consists of the mesh-like system of neurons that govern the function of the gastrointestinal system. Sometimes referred to as the "second brain," it has around 100 million neurons and is in charge of peristalsis, the snake like contraction of your GI tract and the eliciting of certain enzymes to help in digestion. Just like all the other nerves we have talked about, they communicate with each other via neurotransmitters (chemical messengers). Most of these neurotransmitters are identical to the ones found in your CNS such as acetylcholine, dopamine, and serotonin. In fact, more than 90% of the body's serotonin and 50% of the body's dopamine are found hanging out in the enteric nervous system. New and very exciting research is being done now to help understand the importance of this part of us beyond its mechanical functioning.

Sympathetic Nervous System

The sympathetic nervous system is often referred to as the "fight or flight" system. It really gets a bad rap in our yoga culture, being blamed for every illness and evil that arises, but I have to say that in my opinion, except for orgasm (sorry Mom and Dad), it's the coolest thing our nervous system can do! This is what I like to call our "super hero" system. It is activated during stress or great danger, and through a coordinated set of physiological responses, it allows us to fight or flee a situation. This response has helped to keep us around for hundreds of thousands of years. Its nerves mostly originate and are arranged in the thoraco-lumbar region and innervate the organs and glands. If you have ever heard of the stories of the tiny mother who was able to lift a car off her trapped child, or the unbelievable stories of survival against the odds, this is due to the chemical bath of the sympathetic nervous system activation. The problem is that we do tend to activate this system when there is no immediate danger around. Our very powerful and complicated minds can create "danger" and turn on the drip of these chemicals over one hundred times a day, according to some research. While sometimes this might feel useful to us to get "in the zone," we are really not made to marinate in these chemicals. We have evolved to be able to get a big rush of these chemicals to help us, say, run away from a tiger, but after we fought the tiger and won, or ran like the wind in the other direction and reached safety, we were allowed to metabolize the chemicals quickly to return back to our resting state. This constant nudging of our sympathetic nervous system creates what I term a "slow drip," or an "orange alert" response.

If you remember, President George Bush and his administration created a lovely, rainbow-colored chart to tell us how terrified we should be at any given moment, with red being *"holy cow, we are all doomed,"* and blue being *"peace and love and kissing kittens."* The problem is, we were always, and in fact still are on orange alert. This indicates that we should always be slightly terrified with no information or release to be found. This will very literally wear down the tissues of the body. Let me say that again so you know I'm serious: this isn't "crunchy granola yoga talk," you will LITERALLY wear down the tissues of the body! When we are on orange alert in our nervous system and marinating in this slow chemical drip, we will have a lower threshold for activation, greater reactivity, and when we really need this system, it will be less available to give the big bang of chemical reaction. Think of the last time your boss or partner asked you to do something small, but something that you really didn't care to do. If he had asked you on a calm, restful day you might have obliged without fuss, but if he had asked you after a stressful week of work, you might have exploded into a tirade of arm waving and expletives. This has a chemical basis. Let's take a look at what chemically happens to you when, say, an actual tiger is coming after you, and then why it might not be a good idea if these chemicals stuck around on orange alert.

TIGER: Activating stress hormones like adrenaline are produced and released into the system. Adrenaline is like having a few cups of coffee in that it perks you up and allows to you move and make things happen quicker.

ORANGE ALERT: Almost like having too many cups of coffee in your day, this can lead to shakiness, anxiety conditions and insomnia.

TIGER: Glucose, fats, and proteins are released from the fatty tissues, liver, and your muscles. In these situations, your body doesn't have the time or luxury to wait for you to digest the burrito you ate for lunch, so almost like a tiny pickpocket, it steals the food from wherever it can to give you the fuel that you will need.

ORANGE ALERT: With all of the glucose, fats, and proteins running around your system, your chances of getting Type 2 diabetes and metabolic syndrome X are increased. The pickpocket is also slyly stealing the nutrition needed for the muscles to do their job, which could lead to muscle wasting.

TIGER: Your breathing rate and volume will increase and your bronchial passages will dilate to give your body the oxygen it needs.

ORANGE ALERT: This actually leads to something called paradoxical inhibited breathing pattern. This is where the breath gets very shallow, you unintentionally hold the breath, or fight its very nature by fighting the lowering of the diaphragm (sucking the belly in as you inhale and pushing the belly out on the exhale).

TIGER: Your heart rate and blood pressure will rise and the deep arteries to the skeletal muscles will dilate. This allows all of this fuel and oxygen to get where it needs to go faster and more efficiently.

ORANGE ALERT: Sustained high blood pressure puts us at an increased risk of circulatory disorders.

TIGER: Your metabolic rate will increase because now that you have all of this oxygen and fuel transported to the tissues that need it, the cells need to metabolize it faster to make it available to you right now.

ORANGE ALERT: This metabolic increase is not sustained and actually can lead to weight gain. When the body senses danger, it tends to shut down the metabolizing process as if it senses famine and it's not sure when its going to be fed again.

TIGER: To prevent hemorrhaging, the more superficial blood vessels will constrict and clotting substances will be produced and released in case the tiger actually gets you. Some aspects of your immune system like inflammation are enhanced just in case you may need them.

ORANGE ALERT: This again has been linked to an increased risk for circulatory disease and autoimmune disorders.

TIGER: Your senses are heightened. The pupils will dilate and your brain activity will increase. This helps you see and interpret the situation quicker and more clearly to determine how to get out of there. The muscles will tighten and begin to contract to prepare for the action.

ORANGE ALERT: If your muscles are constantly being told to prepare for action, this can and does lead to chronic muscle tension and pain. If your mind is racing even no actual threat exists, this can lead to insomnia.

TIGER: Because your body is doing all of these cool super hero things, to be more efficient, the functions that aren't really necessary in that moment temporally go "offline." At that moment, you don't really need to worry about digesting the burrito you had for lunch, or your egg/sperm maturation, or even your long-term immune function or memory consolidation - there's a tiger in front of you, for goodness' sake!

ORANGE ALERT: I think you see where I'm going with this. The reproductive, digestive, and immune systems are really important systems, and it's like your body constantly whispers to them that they're not really needed right now. This leads to chronic digestive disorders, infertility, and a suppressed immune system.

TIGER: Over a longer period of time, other stress hormones like cortisol are produced and released to help with the inflammation that may have occurred.

ORANGE ALERT: Your brain and body really are not meant to marinate in a cortisol bath, and this is shown to be linked to depression, a suppressed immune system, and increased fat storage.

Are you completely stressed out now? Well, don't worry, your fantastic body has a shut off valve for this chemical drip. After the tiger attack, you are biologically compelled to reach out for comfort and safety in your social groups. As you reach safety, your body starts to produce oxytocin. Oxytocin is one of your body's hormones that helps to form trust and pair bonds and is sometimes termed the "cuddling hormone." Your body will start to produce a small amount of this hormone which will compel you to reach out to someone (physically and emotionally) and say something like, *"Hey, there was a tiger! It was so scary!"* The physical and emotional care from your loved ones will help turn the oxytocin faucet on stronger, which will shut off the sympathetic nervous system activation. It will also help you to turn on the parasympathetic nervous system, or the "rest and digest" system where all of your body's housekeeping activities can be maintained...ahh.

Parasympathetic Nervous System

The parasympathetic nervous system is sometimes referred to as the "rest and digest" system, and its activation is coined as the relaxation response. The relaxation response is a coordinated set of physiological changes that promotes your body's long-term projects like reproduction, digestion, growth and repair, fighting disease, and learning. Its nerves mostly originate from the brain stem and sacral regions (craniosacral) and travel to a lot of the same organs and glands as the sympathetic branch, but, for the most part, will have the opposite response when activated.

There are many ways we specifically try to activate the parasympathetic nervous system in our yoga practice. Like money in the bank accrues interest over time (or so I've heard), repeated practice of relaxation techniques will improve their effectiveness. At first, you may have to put in a lot of time to have a profound relaxation response, but even the attempt alone is often enough to turn it on.

Some ways to elicit the relaxation response:

Muscle relaxation/muscle exhaustion: The conscious letting go of muscle tension, or by perhaps exhausting the muscles so they have no choice but to let go, triggers the body to relax.

Inversions, or reclining with the head below the heart: Being bipeds, our head usually exists above our heart. For this reason, we have a gorgeous and complicated arterial system to fight against gravity to supply the hungry brain with what it needs, but a stingy venous system to return deoxygenated blood back from the head to the lungs and heart for recycling. Our veins are also quite stretchy and can hold a tremendous amount of blood volume. When we lower the head below our heart, our blood pressure to our head increases due to the new pull of gravity. We have little barroreceptors or "thermostats" in the arteries that lead to the head that, sensing this increase, will tell the heart and lungs to slow down as to not overwhelm the system. So, by hanging out in a peaceful inversion, our blood pressure and breathing will slow down, helping to elicit the relaxation response.

Extending the exhale/Slow breathing: Slow deepening of the breath helps to trigger the vagus nerve, a major parasympathetic nerve. Every time you inhale, your heart speeds up a tiny bit, and every time you exhale, your heartbeat slows down. The old advice from your mom to take a deep breath, or the pestering of your yoga teacher to slow down your exhale are actually ways to help relax.

Silence or repetitive sounds: Ok, this one is slightly subjective. The repetitive sounds from your yoga teacher's Sounds of the Rainforest CD could drive you nuts, but repetitive sounds and movements are said to help elicit the relaxation response. The lack of emotional and mental arousal also are said to help, but as we know, that's easier said than done.

Perceived physical safety: All of the deep breathing and hanging upside down while listening to your favorite Yanni tunes will not have a profound effect on you if there is a tiger pacing outside of your door! Your house, so to speak, must be put in order, because this relaxation response is strongly influenced by all aspects of your life.

Final Thoughts

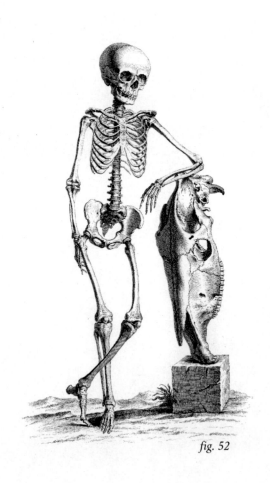

fig. 52

"No one can stand in these solitudes unmoved, and not feel that there is more in man than the mere breath of his body."

- CHARLES DARWIN, THE VOYAGE OF THE BEAGLE

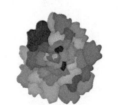

"What is the ultimate truth about ourselves? Various answers suggest themselves. We are a bit of stellar matter gone wrong. We are physical machinery-puppets that strut and talk and laugh and die as the hand of time pulls the strings beneath. But there is one elementary inescapable answer. We are the one which asks the question."

- SIR ARTHUR EDDINGTON

The Beginning, the middle and the end

All my classes and workshops begin with the Sanskrit chant that was given to me by my first teacher.

Guru Brahma
Guru Vishnu
Guru Devo Maheshvarah
Guru Sakshat Param Brahma
Tasmai Shri Gurave Namaha

It is a lovely and profound chant which I translate as the following:

The beginnings are our teacher. The start of something new, coming into a posture and even inhaling are an opportunity to learn the truth of who we are.

The experience of right now in the present moment can be our teacher. The trials and tribulations, the ups and downs, the sustaining of the breath or posture are opportunities to understand the truth of who we are.

The endings of things are our teacher. The ending of a job or relationship, the exhale and coming out of a posture are all opportunities to realize the truth of who we are.

There is a teacher that is nearby. Everyone around you is a teacher that can help to illuminate the truth of who you are.

There is a teacher who is indescribable and beyond all form.

I offer all of my efforts to the teacher. Everything, everyone and every moment become an opportunity to learn about ourselves.

This is just the beginning. My hope is that after this introduction to your body you are excited to continue learning and asking questions. Even after many years of studying the body, I am amazed at how my perception and understanding continues to shift. My first attempt to understand the body came from books and two dimensional pictures. It was only after I started to work with real bodies in yoga classes and anatomy labs did I come to realize how utterly unique we are. Looking at real bodies also begins to unveil the truth that everything is interconnected, interwoven and interdependent. While it may be helpful to label individual body parts for study the reality is nothing can be separated. Many of the separate tissues that we label in the body were arbitrary lines drawn by anatomists. Like looking at a map of the United States of America, some state borders seem to make sense. Mountain ranges and rivers, like tissue function and action, create easy to define borders but taking a larger view we see that it is truly all connected.

The celebration of our differences, the ever shifting transient nature of body, mind and emotion can lead us back to the recollection and reuniting with the part of us that is unbound and pure potential. When we recognize that part of us it then becomes easier to recognize that in others. This practice ultimately leads to the remembrance and honoring of our connectedness.

I always end my classes by saying,

Om Bolo Shri Sat Guru Bhagavan Ki Jai

Truth is the real teacher

Namaste

About the author

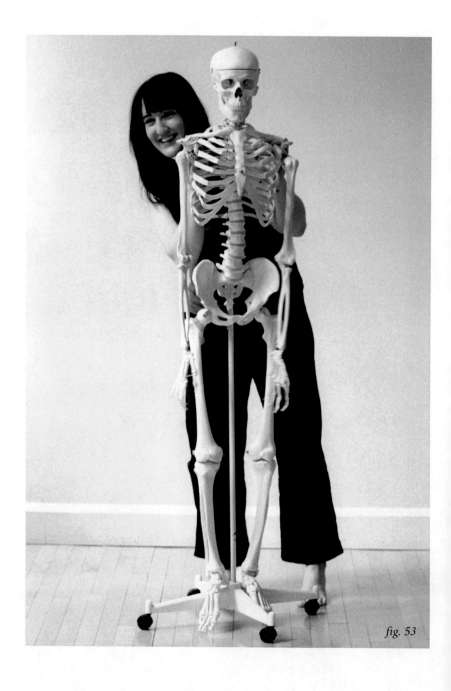

fig. 53

Kristin Leal

Kristin's teachings are infused with the miracle of the human body and the liberating potential of movement. Her unique and dynamic voice makes her classes a powerful blend of strong anatomical alignment and intense vinyasa flow. She is the creator of the Kaya Yoga 200- and 300- hour teacher training - graduating thousands of students since 2005 - and leads workshops around the world. In love with how esoteric anatomy links so effortlessly to Western anatomy, her MetaAnatomy TM trainings blend serious scientific knowledge with a sense of humor and a deep connection to the divine within us all.

Her teachers have included Sharon Gannon, David Life, Katchie Ananda, Adrienne Burke, Rodney Yee, and Betsey Downing and their beautiful teachings, along with her students, continue to inspire her every day. Since 2006, she has been working with and studying under the teacher Yogiraj Alan Finger of ISHTA yoga and has helped this yogi master translate his teachings to help create his 300 - hour and ISHTA marma point teacher training. A licensed massage therapist since 1995 (Swedish Institute of Massage), she also holds certifications in Reiki, Thai Massage, Neuromuscular and myofascial release, and is the co-author of the book "The Yoga Fan" (reviewed as "an indispensable guide for the serious yoga student.") and author of MetaAnatomy TM Volume 1. She is currently working on her third book, MetaAnatomy TM Volume 2, due out soon.

For more information check out:

www.kristinleal.com
www.metaanatomy.com
www.thebeautyinthebones.tumblr.com
www.facebook/metaanatomy.com

Bibliography

Fig 1 - Vinci, Leonardo da. Anatomy and Physiology for Nurses. New York, NY: The Macmillan Company, 1907. Retrieved December 2013, from http://etc.usf.edu/clipart/plants/live_oak_1.html

Fig 2 - Photo by Dmitriy Shironosov. Retrieved December 2013, from http://www.dreamstime.com/

Fig 3 - Photo by Susan Berman. Retrieved December 2013, from www.flickr.com/photos/8773000@N08/8066266815/in/set-72157631719364779

Fig 4 - Chancellor, William E. Standard Short Courses for Evening Schools. New York: American Book Company, 1911. 250. http://etc.usf.edu/clipart/44000/44014/44014_skeleton.htm

Fig 5 - Gray, Henry. Gray's Anatomy. New York NY: Bounty, 1901. N. 51. Fig. 22. Print

Steele, Joel Dorman Hygienic Physiology. New York, NY: A. S. Barnes & Company, 1888. Retrieved December 2013, from http://etc.usf.edu/clipart/50600/50668/50668_thorax.htm

Cunningham, D.J. Textbook of Anatomy. New York, NY: William Wood and Co., 1903. Retrieved December 2013, from http://etc.usf.edu/clipart/54600/54655/54655_skull.htm, http://etc.usf.edu/clipart/54600/54654/54654_hyoid.htm, http://etc.usf.edu/clipart/56600/56617/56617_tympanic.htm

Fig 6 - How to Draw and Paint. New York: Excelsior Publishing House. 131, 141, 145 Retrieved December 2013, from http://etc.usf.edu/clipart/28800/28895/shoulder_28895.htm, http://etc.usf.edu/clipart/28900/28903/bones_28903.htm, http://etc.usf.edu/clipart/28900/28910/leg3_28910.htm

Cunningham, D.J. Textbook of Anatomy. New York, NY: William Wood and Co., 1903. Retrieved December 2013, from http://etc.usf.edu/clipart/54600/54677/54677_pelvis.htm

Kimber, Diana C. Anatomy and Physiology for Nurses. New York, NY: The Macmillan Company, 1907. Retrieved December 2013, from http://etc.usf.edu/clipart/35300/35358/wrist_hand_35358.htm

William Dwight Whitney The Century Dictionary: An Encyclopedic Lexicon of the English Language. New York, NY: The Century Co., 1911. Retrieved December 2013, from http://etc.usf.edu/clipart/62900/62989/62989_foot_bones.htm

Fig 7 - Frank Leslie, The Kingdom of Nature, an Illustrated Museum of the Animal World. Chicage: Thompson & Thomas, 1900. 35 Retrieved December 2013, from http://etc.usf.edu/clipart/23700/23770/skeleton_23770.htmv

Fig 8 - Cunningham, D.J. Textbook of Anatomy. New York, NY: William Wood and Co., 1903. Retrieved December 2013, from http://etc.usf.edu/clipart/55200/55212/55212_joint.htm

Fig 9 - Cunningham, D J, and Arthur Robinson. Cunningham's Text-Book of Anatomy. 4th ed. London: H. Frowde and Hodder & Stoughton, 1914. N. 347, Fig. 320. Print.

Fig 10 - John W. Ritchie Primer of Physiology. New York: World Book Company, 1918. 28 Retrieved December 2013, from http://etc.usf.edu/clipart/19800/19884/armmsclstrc_19884.htm

Fig 11 - Patanjali Kundalini Yoga Care, Joan S. Harrigan, © 2012 Retrieved December 2013, from http://www.authenticmovementjournal.com/wp-content/uploads/2012/01/Patanjali_image.jpg

Fig 12 - Cheselden, William, Osteographia, or The anatomy of the bones.. London: Russell and Wellcome, 1733. 20. Retrived December 2013, http://www.nlm.nih.gov/exhibition/historicalanatomies/Images/1200_pixels/cheselden_t20.jpg

Fig 13 - Gray, Henry. Gray's Anatomy. New York NY: Bounty, 1901. N. 51. Fig. 22. Print

Fig 14 - Gray, Henry. Gray's Anatomy. New York NY: Bounty, 1901. N. 37, 29, 42. Fig. 2, 5, 8. Print.

Fig 15 - Gray, Henry. Gray's Anatomy. New York NY: Lea & Febiger, 1918. N. 288. Fig. 301. Print.

Fig 16 - Gray, Henry. Gray's Anatomy. New York NY: Bounty, 1901. N. 37, 38. Fig. 2, 4. Print.
Gray, Henry. Gray's Anatomy. New York NY: Lea & Febiger, 1918. N.100. Fig. 87. Print.

Fig 17 - Gray, Henry. Gray's Anatomy. New York NY: Bounty, 1901. N. 39. Fig. 5. Print.

Fig 18 - Gray, Henry. Gray's Anatomy. New York NY: Bounty, 1901. N. 42. Fig. 8. Print.

Fig 19 - Gray, Henry. Gray's Anatomy. New York NY: Bounty, 1901. N. 37, 38. Fig. 2, 4. Print.
Gray, Henry. Gray's Anatomy. New York NY: Lea & Febiger, 1918. N.109. Fig. 97. Print.

Fig 20 - Gray, Henry. Gray's Anatomy. New York NY: Bounty, 1901. N. 50. Fig. 21. Print.

Fig 21 - Gray, Henry. Gray's Anatomy. New York NY: Bounty, 1901. N. 344. Fig. 214. Print.

Fig 22 - Gray, Henry. Gray's Anatomy. New York NY: Bounty, 1901. N. 318, 333. Fig. 202, 210. Print.

Fig 23 - Gray, Henry. Gray's Anatomy. New York NY: Bounty, 1901. N. 358, 360. Fig. 218, 219. Print.

Fig 24 - Cheselden, William, Osteographia, or The anatomy of the bones.. London: Russell and Wellcome, 1733. 30. Retrived December 2013, http://www.nlm.nih.gov/exhibition/historicalanatomies/Images/1200_pixels/cheselden_t30.jpg

Fig 25 - Gray, Henry. Gray's Anatomy. New York NY: Bounty, 1901. N. 178. Fig. 122. Print.

Fig 26 - Gray, Henry. Gray's Anatomy. New York NY: Bounty, 1901. N. 179, 180. Fig. 123, 124. Print.

Fig 27 - Gray, Henry. Gray's Anatomy. New York NY: Bounty, 1901. N. 184. Fig. 126. Print.

Fig 28 - Gray, Henry. Gray's Anatomy. New York NY: Bounty, 1901. N. 193. Fig. 133. Print.

Fig 29 - Gray, Henry. Gray's Anatomy. New York NY: Bounty, 1901. N. 200. Fig. 137. Print.

Fig 30 - Gray, Henry. Gray's Anatomy. New York NY: Bounty, 1901. N. 420. Fig. 253. Print.

Fig 31 - Gray, Henry. Gray's Anatomy. New York NY: Bounty, 1901. N. 256. Fig. 428. Print.

Fig 32 - The Division of General Surgery Manual of Surgical Anatomy. Washington, DC: Medical Departments U.S. Army and Navy, 1918. Retrieved December 2013, from http://etc.usf.edu/cli-part/52800/52854/52854_thigh.htm

Fig 33 - Gray, Henry. Gray's Anatomy. New York NY: Bounty, 1901. N. 424. Fig. 254. Print.

Fig 34 - Cunningham, D J, and Arthur Robinson. Cunningham's Text-Book of Anatomy. 4th ed. London: H. Frowde and Hodder & Stoughton, 1914. N. 380. Fig. 426. Print.

Fig 35 - Gray, Henry. Gray's Anatomy. New York NY: Bounty, 1901. N. 372, 374. Fig. 225, 227. Print.

Fig 36 - Gray, Henry. Gray's Anatomy. New York NY: Bounty, 1901. N. 276. Fig. 185. Print.
Gray, Henry. Gray's Anatomy. New York NY: Lea & Febiger, 1918. N.342. Fig. 348. Print.

Fig 37 - Gray, Henry. Gray's Anatomy. New York NY: Bounty, 1901. N. 437, 439. Fig. 259, 260. Print.

Fig 38 - Gray, Henry. Gray's Anatomy. New York NY: Lea & Febiger, 1918. N 100. Fig. 87. Print.

Fig 39 - Gewehr, Felipe - Traced Skeleton. Retrieved December 2013, from http://felipe-gewehr.deviantart.com/art/Traced-Skeleton-399019195*Fig 40* - Gray, Henry. Gray's Anatomy. New York NY: Bounty, 1901. N. 138, 139. Fig. 94, 95. Print.

Gray, Henry. Gray's Anatomy. New York NY: Lea & Febiger, 1918. N 207. Fig. 205. Print.

Fig 41- Gray, Henry. Gray's Anatomy. New York NY: Bounty, 1901. N. 136. Fig. 92. Print.

Fig 42 - Gray, Henry. Gray's Anatomy. New York NY: Bounty, 1901. N. 145, 151. Fig. 97, 100. Print.

Fig 43 - Gray, Henry. Gray's Anatomy. New York NY: Bounty, 1901. N. 159. Fig. 104. Print.
Henry Gray Anatomy Descriptive and Applied. New York, NY: Lea & Febiger, 1913. Retrieved December 2013, from http://etc.usf.edu/cli-part/24200/24240/foot_skeleto_24240.htm

Fig 44 - Gray, Henry. Gray's Anatomy. New York NY: Bounty, 1901. N. 385. Fig. 232. Print.

Fig 45 - Gray, Henry. Gray's Anatomy. New York NY: Bounty, 1901. N. 379. Fig. 229. Print.

Fig 46 - Gray, Henry. Gray's Anatomy. New York NY: Bounty, 1901. N. 380. Fig. 230. Print.

Fig 47 - Gray, Henry. Gray's Anatomy. New York NY: Bounty, 1901. N. 338. Fig. 213. Print.

Fig 48 - Albert F. Blaisedell Our bodies and How We Live. Boston: Ginn &, 1904. 162 Retrieved December 2013, from http://etc.usf.edu/cli-part/15400/15498/lungs_15498.htm

Fig 49 - Gray, Henry. Gray's Anatomy. New York NY: Bounty, 1901. N. 353. Fig. 216. Print.

Fig 50 - Gray, Henry. Gray's Anatomy. New York NY: Bounty, 1901. N. 974. Fig. 538. Print.

Fig 51- Retrieved December 2013, from http://wallpaperswide.com/nervous_system-wallpapers.html

Fig 52 - Cheselden, William, Osteographia, or The anatomy of the bones. London: Russell and Wellcome, 1733. 33. Retrived December 2013, http://www.nlm.nih.gov/exhibition/historicalanatomies/Images/1200_pixels/cheselden_t33.jpg

Fig 53 - Photo by Jenean Nanette.

Made in the USA
San Bernardino, CA
24 October 2016